Fractures of the Tibia

Nirmal C. Tejwani

Editor

Fractures of the Tibia

A Clinical Casebook

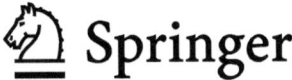 Springer

Editor
Nirmal C. Tejwani, MD
NYU Langone Medical Center
Hospital for Joint Diseases
New York, NY, USA

ISBN 978-3-319-21773-4   ISBN 978-3-319-21774-1   (eBook)
DOI 10.1007/978-3-319-21774-1

Library of Congress Control Number: 2015956210

Springer Cham Heidelberg New York Dordrecht London

Printed on acid-free paper

Springer International Publishing AG Switzerland is part of Springer Science+Business Media (www.springer.com)

This book is dedicated to my wife Mona and my two lovely daughters Ruchi and Rhea, as it would not have been possible without their support and encouragement.

Preface

Tibia fractures are commonly treated with internal fixation in a variety of ways using different implants and techniques. This is based on fracture type and location, soft tissue status, implant availability, as well as surgeon experience. With the spectrum of injuries ranging from intra-articular fractures to segmental shaft fractures and complex combinations of injuries, the treatment methods vary widely. Fractures of the tibial plateau are treated in a staged manner similar to pilon fractures, primarily for soft tissue management. The use of internal or external fixation is described using actual cases as treated by the authors.

The purpose of this book is to give the readers case examples of different tibia fractures from the plateau to the pilon and their treatment options. This book is entirely case based and uses clinical case scenarios and attempts to put the reader in the surgeon's shoes. Each case aims to illustrate different options for treatment with the authors' rationale and follow-up with outcomes of the options used in treatment. The goal is not to substitute knowledge learning from textbooks or journals but to provide clinical examples elucidating the translation of theory to practice.

The reader must be aware that not all of these treatment options may be applicable to all situations, but will hopefully make you aware of the same.

The creation of this book would not have been possible without the conceptual insight of Kristopher Spring (editor, Clinical Medicine) and the logistical support of Brian Halm (development editor), both at Springer. Much gratitude is owed to them for their professionalism and engagement that resulted in the timely execution of the project.

New York, NY, USA   Nirmal C. Tejwani

Contents

Part II   Treatment of Tibia Shaft Fractures

Part III   Treatment of Open Tibia Fractures

Part IV   Treatment of Distal Tibia Articular Fractures

Contributors

Pramod Achan, FRCS Trauma and Orthopaedics, The Royal London Hospital, Bart's Health NHS Trust, London, UK

Jaimo Ahn, MD Department of Orthopaedic Surgery, University of Pennsylvania, Philadelphia, PA, USA

Michael T. Archdeacon, MD Department of Orthopaedic Surgery, University of Cincinnati, College of Medicine, Cincinnati, OH, USA

Jennifer M. Bauer, MD Vanderbilt University, Nashville, TN, USA

John Buza, MD Department of Orthopaedic Surgery, Hospital for Joint Diseases, NYU Langone Medical Center, New York, NY, USA

Lisa K. Cannada, MD Division of Orthopaedic Surgery, Saint Louis University, St. Louis, MD, USA

Natalie Casemyr, MD Division of Orthopaedic Trauma, Yale School of Medicine, New Haven, CT, USA

Cory A. Collinge, MD Orthopedic Trauma, Harris Methodist Fort Worth Hospital/John Peter Smith Orthopedic Surgery Residency, Fort Worth, TX, USA

Aaron T. Creek, MD Department of Orthopaedic Surgery, Greenville Health System, Greenville, SC, USA

Roy I. Davidovitch, MD Department of Orthopaedic Surgery, NYU Langone- Hospital for Joint Diseases, New York, NY, USA

Huw Edwards, MD Trauma and Orthopaedics, The Royal London Hospital, Bart's Health NHS Trust, London, UK

Kenneth Egol, MD Division of Trauma Service, Department of Orthopaedic Surgery, Hospital for Joint Diseases, NYU Langone Medical Center, New York, NY, USA

Juan Favela, MD Harvard University, Boston, MA, USA Orthopedic Specialty Associates, Fort Worth, TX, USA

David K. Galos, MD Division of Orthopaedic Trauma, Department of Orthopaedic Surgery, NYU Langone-Hospital for Joint Diseases, New York, NY, USA

David Hak, MD, MBA, FACS Division of Orthopaedic Trauma, Denver Health Medical Center, Denver, Colorado, USA

Mark Hake, MD Division of Orthopaedic Trauma, University of Michigan, Ann Arbor, MI, USA

Mitchel B. Harris, MD Harvard Medical School Orthopaedic Trauma Initiative, Boston, MA, USA Department of Orthopaedics, Brigham and Women's Hospital, Boston, MA, USA

Marilyn Heng, MD Harvard Medical School Orthopaedic Trauma Initiative, Boston, MA, USA Department of Orthopaedics, Brigham and Women's Hospital, Boston, MA, USA Department of Orthopaedics, Massachusetts General Hospital, Boston, MA, USA

D. S. Horwitz, MD Department of Orthopaedic Surgery, Geisinger Medical Center, Danville, PA, USA

A. Alex Jahangir, MD Division of Orthopaedic Trauma, Department of Orthopaedic Surgery and Rehabilitation, Vanderbilt University Medical Center, Nashville, TN, USA

Kyle J. Jeray, MD Department of Orthopaedic Surgery, Greenville Health System, Greenville, SC, USA

Charlie Jowett, MD Trauma and Orthopaedics, The Royal London Hospital, Bart's Health NHS Trust, London, UK

Rafael Kakazu, MD Department of Orthopaedic Surgery, University of Cincinnati, College of Medicine, Cincinnati, OH, USA

Namdar Kazemi, MD Department of Orthopaedic Surgery, University of Cincinnati, College of Medicine, Cincinnati, OH, USA

H. Kempegowda, MD Department of Orthopaedic Surgery, Geisinger Medical Center, Danville, PA, USA

Elliott J. Kim, MD Division of Orthopaedic Trauma, Department of Orthopaedic Surgery and Rehabilitation, Vanderbilt University Medical Center, Nashville, TN, USA

Sanjit A. Konda, MD Department of Orthopaedic Surgery, NYU Langone Medical Center, NYU Hospital for Joint Diseases, New York, NY, USA
Division of Orthopaedic Trauma, Jamaica Hospital Medical Center, New York, NY, USA

James Lachman, MD Department of Orthopaedic Surgery, Temple University, Philadelphia, PA, USA

Frank A. Liporace, MD Division of Orthopaedic Trauma, Department of Orthopaedic Surgery, NYU Hospital for Joint Diseases, New York, NY, USA

Cyril Mauffrey, MD, FACS Division of Orthopaedic Trauma,
Denver Health Medical Center, Denver, Colorado, USA

Toni M. McLaurin, MD Department of Orthopaedics, NYU
Hospital for Joint Diseases, New York, NY, USA

William Min, MD The Hughston Clinic at Gwinnett
Medical Center, Lawrenceville, GA, USA

Hassan R. Mir, MD University of South Florida,
Tampa, FL, USA

Edward Perez, MD Department of Orthopaedic Trauma,
Campbell Clinic Orthopaedics, Memphis, TN, USA

Saqib Rehman, MD Department of Orthopaedic Surgery,
Temple University, Philadelphia, PA, USA

Henry Claude Sagi, MD Orthopaedic Trauma Service,
Florida Orthopaedic Institute, North Tampa, FL, USA

Daniel N. Segina, MD Orthopaedic Trauma, Holmes
Regional Trauma Center, Melbourne, FL, USA
University of Central Florida College of Medicine,
Orlando, FL, USA

Milan K. Sen, MD Division of Orthopedic Surgery,
Orthopedic Trauma Jacobi Medical Center, Albert Einstein
College of Medicine Orthopedic Trauma, Wrist, and
Elbow Surgeon, Gotham City Orthopedics LLC, New York,
NY, USA

Anjan R. Shah, MD Orthopaedic Trauma Service, Florida
Orthopaedic Institute, North Tampa, FL, USA

A. A. Tawari, MD Department of Orthopaedic Surgery,
Geisinger Medical Center, Danville, PA, USA

Kostas Triantafillou, MD Department of Orthopaedic
Trauma, Campbell Clinic Orthopaedics, Memphis, TN, USA

Michael J. Weaver, MD Harvard Medical School
Orthopaedic Trauma Initiative, Boston, MA, USA
Department of Orthopaedics, Brigham and Women's
Hospital, Boston, MA, USA

Philip R. Wolinksy, MD Orthopedic Trauma Service,
Department of Orthopedic Surgery, University of California
at Sacramento Medical Center, Sacramento, CA, USA

Chase C. Woodward, MD Department of Orthopaedic
Surgery, University of Pennsylvania, Philadelphia, PA, USA

Richard S. Yoon, MD Division of Orthopaedic Trauma,
Department of Orthopaedic Surgery, NYU Hospital for
Joint Diseases, New York, NY, USA

Part I
Treatment of Proximal Tibia Articular Fractures

Chapter 1
Schatzker I/II Tibia Plateau Fracture

Sanjit A. Konda

Clinical History

The patient is a 39-year-old female involved in a low-speed motor vehicle accident in which her car was rear-ended and then fishtailed into an embankment. On arrival to the emergency department, her Glasgow Coma Scale was 15, and she was complaining of bilateral knee pain. Plain radiographs of bilateral knees demonstrated split-depression fractures of bilateral lateral tibial plateaus (Shatzker II). Computed tomography scans of both knees were obtained, and the diagnosis was confirmed. The patient was then taken to the operating room the same day for operative fixation of bilateral tibial plateaus (Figs. 1.1 and 1.2).

S.A. Konda
Department of Orthopaedic Surgery, NYU Langone Medical Center,
NYU Hospital for Joint Diseases, 301 E 17th St, Suite 1402,
New York, NY 10003, USA

Division of Orthopaedic Trauma, Jamaica Hospital Medical Center,
301 E 17th St, Suite 1402, New York, NY 10003, USA
e-mail: Sanjith.konda@nyumc.org

© Springer International Publishing Switzerland 2016
N.C. Tejwani (ed.), *Fractures of the Tibia: A Clinical Casebook*,
DOI 10.1007/978-3-319-21774-1_1

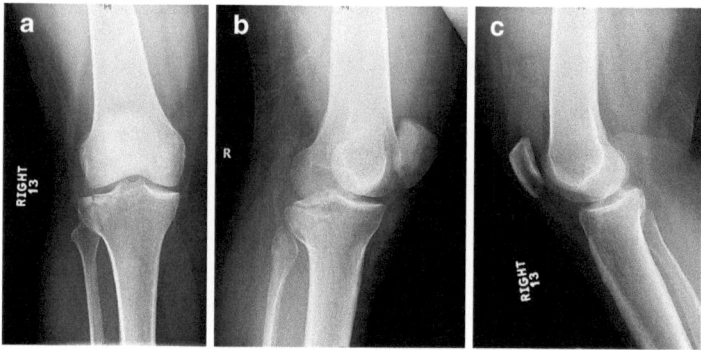

Fig. 1.1 (a–c) Injury films of the right knee. Anteroposterior, oblique, and lateral plane radiographs demonstrating a Shatzker II tibial plateau fracture

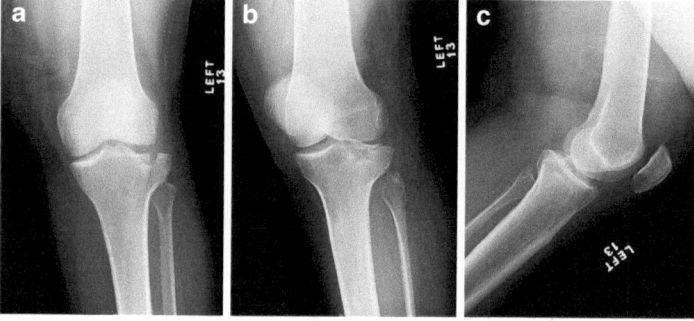

Fig. 1.2 (a–c) Injury films of the left knee. Anteroposterior, oblique, and lateral plain radiographs demonstrating a Shatzker II tibial plateau fracture

Treatment Considerations/Planning/Tests

Operative treatment of Shatzker 1 and 2 tibial plateau fractures is indicated if there is

1. Articular surface step-off >2 mm or
2. >10° valgus instability of the knee

Physical examination focuses on the evaluation of valgus instability and attention to the soft-tissue envelope of the knee. The presence of blisters around the knee indicates significant underlying

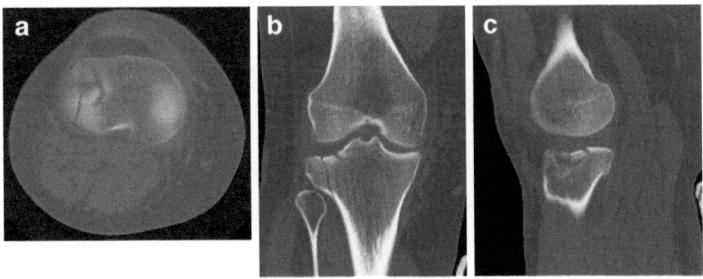

Fig. 1.3 (**a–c**) Injury-computed tomography scan of the right knee. Axial, coronal, and sagittal cuts demonstrating a Shatzker II tibial plateau fracture

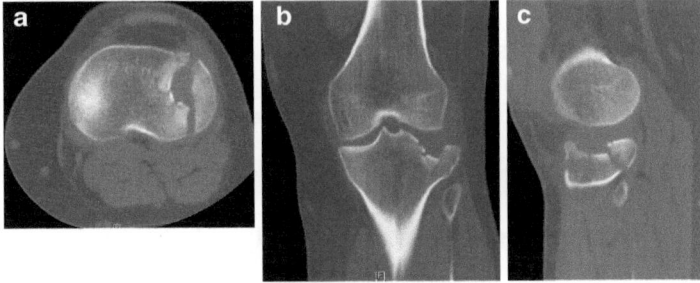

Fig. 1.4 (**a–c**) Injury-computed tomography scan of the left knee. Axial, coronal, and sagittal cuts demonstrating a Shatzker II tibial plateau fracture

soft-tissue injury, and surgery should be delayed until the blisters have re-epithelialized, often between 7 and 14 days.

External fixation of Shatzker 1 and 2 tibial plateau fractures is rarely indicated, as the medial plateau of the tibia is intact providing axial stability to the knee joint. Splinting in a bulky Jones-type dressing and a knee immobilizer is typically sufficient to stabilize the fracture and soft tissues.

Computed tomography scan of the knee should be obtained to further delineate the fracture pattern and aid in preoperative planning (Figs. 1.3 and 1.4).

Preoperative planning entails determining:

1. The location of the depressed articular surface fragments
2. If the sagittal fracture line will allow access to the depressed articular surface

If the depressed articular surface is not accessible by opening the lateral plateau through the sagittal fracture line, then plans should be made to create a lateral cortical window and elevate the articular surface with a bone tamp.

Timing of Surgery

Low-energy Shatzker 1 or 2 fractures (typical fall from standing or low-speed vehicular injuries) generally have little injury to the soft-tissue envelope of the knee and can undergo operative fixation immediately. However, higher energy fractures have moderate to severe swelling at the knee, and surgical incisions should be delayed until the soft-tissue swelling has subsided (1–2 weeks). In the interim, patients should be made NWB and placed into a well-padded knee immobilizer to limit motion at the knee.

Intraoperative Tips and Tricks for Reduction/ Fixation

Utilization of a sterile bump (or nonsterile bump under the sterile drapes) to flex the knee to 30° allows for improved exposure of the joint surface as well as ease of obtaining lateral fluoroscopy views.

A submeniscal arthrotomy should be performed in all cases to directly visualize the joint surface. Tag sutures (#1 vicryl) should be placed into the meniscus for later repair to the lateral plate. A femoral distractor can be used to distract the joint surface with one Schanz pin placed into the distal femur and the other pin placed into the mid-tibia.

The depressed articular surface should be elevated with at least 1–1.5 cm of subchondral bone to allow for sufficient fixation, using raft screws for holding the elevated fragment. Bone void created from elevation of the depressed articular surface should be filled with either cancellous bone chip allograft or calcium phosphate bone substitute to prevent subsequent collapse. Kirschner wires can be placed from lateral to medial directly under the elevated joint surface for provisional fixation. Once the plate is placed onto the lateral aspect of the proximal tibia, a large pelvic reduction clamp can be used to compress the lateral plateau to the intact medial plateau to attain anatomical width of the plateau.

A nonlocking plate is sufficient in good-quality bone as the cortical screws will capture the intact medial plateau and act as rigid rafting screws. The first screw placed through the plate should be just distal to the sagittal split to (1) compress the plate to the tibial shaft and (2) to act as a buttress plate that will prevent distal displacement of the lateral plateau fragment. The second screw placed should be a cortical screw just under the articular surface that will serve to further compress the plate to the lateral tibial plateau. Typically, two cortical shaft screws are sufficient distal fixation for simple Shatzker 1 and 2 fractures (Figs. 1.5 and 1.6).

Postoperative Protocol

Postoperatively, patients are placed into a well-padded knee immobilizer for 1–2 weeks for pain control and to help alleviate postoperative swelling. Prophylactic antibiotics are continued for 24 h postoperatively, and patients are started on chemical prophylaxis for deep vein thrombosis prophylaxis on postoperative day 1.

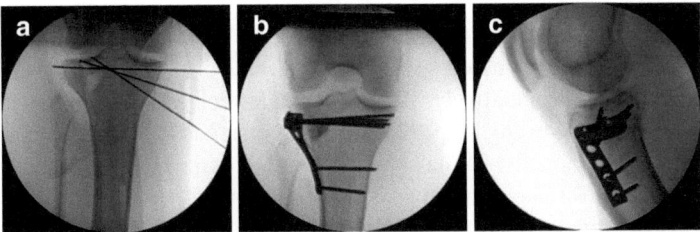

Fig. 1.5 (**a**) Intraoperative radiographs of the right knee demonstrating provisional Kirschner wire fixation of the depressed lateral plateau articular surface. Note the bone void directly below the elevated joint surface. (**b–c**) Final fixation demonstrating restoration of lateral plateau articular congruity. Note the calcium phosphate bone substitute placed into the bone void to provide axial stability to the elevated joint surface

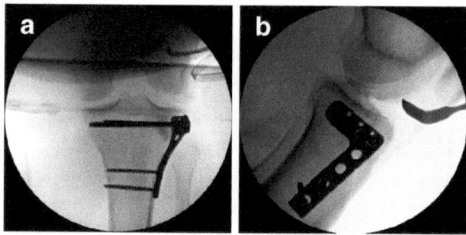

Fig. 1.6 (**a, b**) Intraoperative anteroposterior and lateral radiographs of the left knee demonstrating final fixation construct with restoration of articular congruity and condylar width

Anticoagulation is continued for approximately 4 weeks postoperatively. Early active and passive knee range of motion should be started immediately postoperatively. Isometric quadriceps and hamstring strengthening can be started immediately.

Knee braces in the postoperative period are not necessary if rigid internal fixation is achieved.

Patients remain non-weight-bearing for 3 months postoperatively to allow for healing of the articular surface. At 3 months, patients are advanced to weight-bearing as tolerated. Between 4 and 6 months, patients are allowed to return to full work without restrictions (or full contact sporting activity).

Follow-Up with Union/Complication

Patients are evaluated at 2 weeks, 6 weeks, 3 months, and 6 months, postoperatively. At the second week visit, the surgical incisions are evaluated for healing. Superficial wound dehiscence can be managed with local wound care. Continued wound drainage however should prompt consideration for operative irrigation and debridement of the wound with intraoperative cultures taken to rule out a deep infection. Postoperative radiographs are obtained at the 6-week, 3-month, and 6-month timepoints. If knee flexion remains <90° at 3 months postoperative, then a manipulation of the knee under anesthesia and arthroscopic lysis of adhesions should be performed to aid maximizing knee flexion.

This patient had an uneventful postoperative course. Both left and right knee incisions healed without complications. At

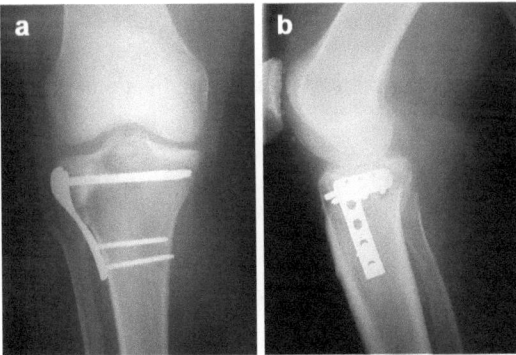

Fig. 1.7 (**a**, **b**) Six-month postoperative plain radiographs of the right knee demonstrating healing of the fracture and maintenance of articular surface congruity

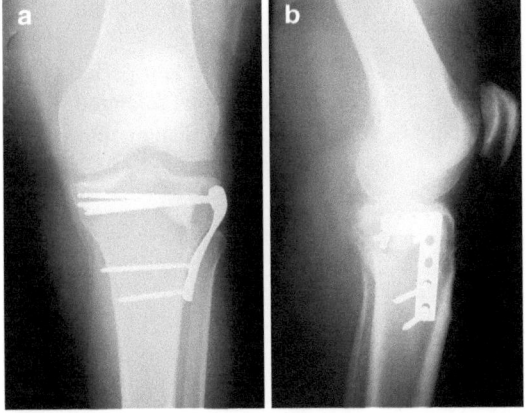

Fig. 1.8 (**a**, **b**) Six-month postoperative plain radiographs of the left knee demonstrating healing of the fracture and maintenance of articular surface congruity

the 3-month postoperative timepoint, she had achieved clinical and radiographic union of both fractures. She had 120° of knee flexion bilaterally. By 6 months postoperatively, the patient was ambulating independently without the use of an assistive device and was ready to return to work without restrictions (Figs. 1.7 and 1.8).

Salient Points/Pearls

- The key to minimizing wound complications is respecting the soft-tissue envelope.
- Low-energy Shatzker I and II fractures can generally be fixed immediately, whereas high-energy fractures require 1–2 weeks of rest and immobilization to allow the soft-tissue swelling to subside.
- A submeniscal arthrotomy on the lateral side is necessary to evaluate the entire meniscus for tears.
- Elevation of the articular surface with a 1–1.5 cm block of subchondral bone allows for "raft screw" placement just under or through the suchondral bone.
- Calcium phosphate bone cement can be used to pack the void left by elevating the joint surface.
- A nonlocking plate with bicortical screw purchase into the proximal tibia is sufficient fixation strength in young adult bone.
- Postoperative protocol should include a period of 3 months of NWB followed by weight-bearing as tolerated. Knee range-of-motion should be initiated as soon as pain allows.

Chapter 2
Schatzker III Tibia Plateau Fracture (with Bone Graft Substitute)

Mark Hake, Natalie Casemyr, Cyril Mauffrey, and David Hak

Short Clinical History

The patient is a 59-year-old female who slipped and fell on ice landing on her left lower extremity. The patient was evaluated in the emergency department, where she complained of isolated left knee pain. Her knee was moderately swollen without open wounds. The compartments of her lower extremity remained soft without evidence of compartment syndrome. Examination found her to be motor and sensory intact. Her past medical and surgical history is noncontributory.

M. Hake (✉)
Division of Orthopaedic Trauma, University of Michigan,
Ann Arbor, Michigan, USA
e-mail: mhake@med.umich.edu

N. Casemyr
Division of Orthopaedic Trauma, Yale School of Medicine,
New Haven, CT, USA

C. Mauffrey • D. Hak
Division of Orthopaedic Trauma, Denver Health Medical Center, Denver,
Colorado, USA

© Springer International Publishing Switzerland 2016   11
N.C. Tejwani (ed.), *Fractures of the Tibia: A Clinical Casebook*,
DOI 10.1007/978-3-319-21774-1_2

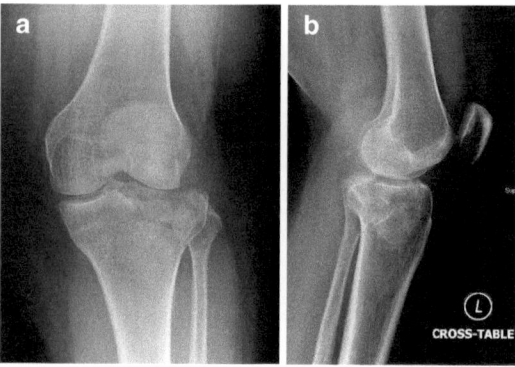

Fig. 2.1 Anteroposterior (**a**) and lateral (**b**) radiographs of the left knee demonstrating a Schatzker III tibial plateau fracture in a 59-year-old female. Note the significant impaction of the articular surface seen on the lateral view

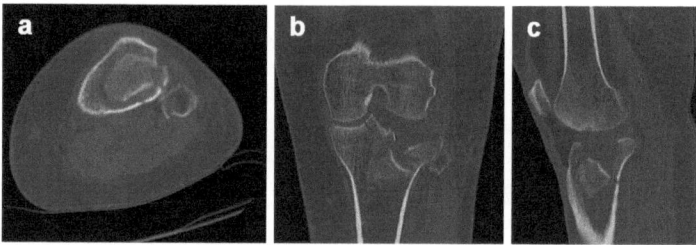

Fig. 2.2 Axial CT cuts through the proximal tibia demonstrating significant lateral plateau involvement of the fracture (**a**). Coronal (**b**) and sagittal (**c**) CT cuts through the proximal tibia demonstrating the location of the depressed fragments within the metaphysis that will require elevation

Plain radiographs showed a Schatzker type III tibial plateau fracture (Fig. 2.1). Multiple articular fragments were depressed into the metaphyseal region. A CT scan was obtained to further evaluate the degree and location of articular depression (Fig. 2.2). The patient's knee was well aligned without significant shortening and was placed in a knee immobilizer, made non-weight-bearing, and sent home with pain control and instructions for strict elevation. She was seen in outpatient clinic prior to her scheduled operative date for evaluation of her soft tissues. Surgery was planned 14 days postinjury. The skin was inspected on the morning of surgery and found to be amenable to safe surgical treatment.

Treatment Considerations/Planning/Tests Needed

Schatzker III tibial plateau fractures are infrequent injuries, but challenging to treat. They are typically seen after lower energy injuries in patients with significant osteoporosis. Because of their association with underlying osteoporosis, they can involve significant displacement and comminution of the articular fragments. Reduction of these displaced fragments can be difficult due to their location within the metaphysis of the tibia and difficulty in visualization of the joint surface.

Surgical treatment goals include anatomic reduction of the articular surface, restoration of the mechanical axis, stable fixation to allow early range of motion, and avoiding infection by preserving the surrounding soft tissues. The degree of depression and ligamentous instability can guide surgical treatment decisions. In general, any injury that causes joint instability or malalignment should be treated operatively to prevent a poor outcome [1]. Joint depression that can be tolerated with conservative management ranges from 4 to 10 mm [2]. A correlation between residual joint step-off and poor outcomes has yet to be shown in the literature [3, 4].

Preoperative planning begins with a thorough history and physical examination. The patient's baseline activity level and medical comorbidities must be considered when developing a treatment strategy. Knee stability and the condition of the soft-tissue envelope determine the imaging needed and timing involved in treatment. Open injuries and compartment syndrome require emergent operative treatment. When there is significant soft tissue injury, external fixation with a knee-spanning construct will allow for soft-tissue healing and maintenance of limb length, until definitive fixation can safely be performed.

Preoperative imaging begins with plain radiographs. AP and lateral views are obtained, along with internal and external rotation oblique views. These oblique views can provide important information about the degree and location of the depressed segments. An AP view with the beam directed 10° caudal shows displacement at the articular surface most clearly. Computed tomography with sagittal and coronal reconstructions has been shown to affect the surgical plan in many cases, as articular depression can be difficult to evaluate on plain radiographs alone [5, 6]. It is crucial to critically examine the CT scan and have a thorough knowledge of the location and orientation of the displaced fragments to have a plan for reduction. MRI of tibial plateau fractures is useful to evaluate for ligamentous or meniscal injury [7, 8]. These injuries, while more common in higher energy injuries, have been shown to occur frequently in all types of tibial plateau fractures. MRI is of little utility once metal implants have been placed due to artifact. If there is concern for ligamentous injury or meniscal injury, then MRI should be obtained preoperatively.

Timing of Surgery

Many Schatzker type III fractures are caused by a low-energy mechanism in osteoporotic bone. While a surgical intervention is best performed in a delayed fashion following high-energy tibial plateau fractures [9], Schatzker type III fractures do not typically require delayed treatment and external fixation. Temporary spanning external fixation can be useful for soft-tissue healing, especially in length-unstable tibial plateau fractures. Avoiding external fixation in the cases when it is not required avoids a trip to the operating room and the increased risks that come with external fixation, such as infection.

Intraoperative Tips and Tricks for Reduction/Fixation

The principles of anatomic articular reduction and stable fixation to allow early range of motion hold true when treating Schatzker III tibial plateau fractures. Because the fracture pattern consists of an isolated central depression, gaining access to the depressed articular fragments presents a particular challenge, as there are no associated fracture planes that can be used to access the articular fragment. A cortical window or intraarticular osteotomy is required to gain access to the fracture fragments.

Positioning and Equipment

The patient is positioned supine on a radiolucent table (Fig. 2.3). A bump placed under the ipsilateral hip helps to control rotation of the hip and expose the lateral aspect of the proximal tibia. A thigh tourniquet is used to improve visualization and minimize blood loss. The patient should be positioned on the lateral side of the table, so that a universal distractor, which can be extremely useful to visualize the lateral joint surface, can be used without interference. Instruments for elevation of the joint surface, such as complete set bone tamps or balloon osteoplasty equipment, will be needed. Osteotomes may be needed for making a cortical window or creating an intraarticular osteotomy (turning a type III pattern into a type II pattern).

Approach

A standard anterolateral approach is used. The incision is centered on Gerdy's tubercle in a "lazy S" fashion (Fig. 2.4). The incision is midaxial at the joint line and moves anteriorly to run parallel and approximately 1–2 cm lateral to the tibial crest. Proximally, the iliotibial band is cut in line with its fibers. The fascia over the anterior compartment is incised and the tibialis anterior gently elevated off the metaphysis using a Cobb elevator. A small cuff of

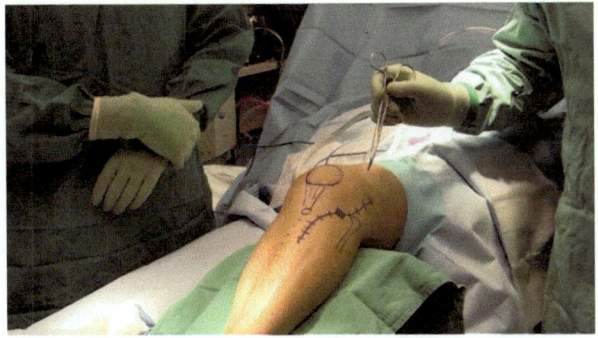

Fig. 2.3 The patient is positioned supine on a radiolucent table. A bump is placed under the ipsilateral hip to allow for improved access to the lateral proximal tibia. A radiolucent triangle can be used to elevate the leg

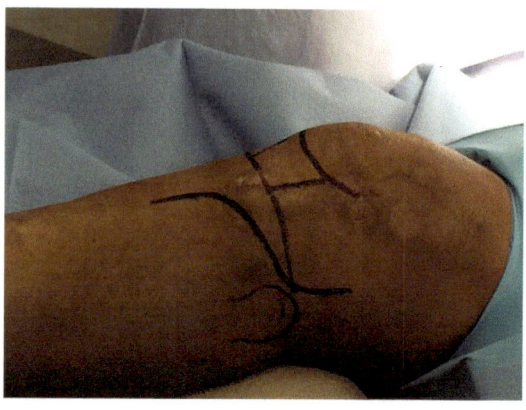

Fig. 2.4 An anterolateral incision is planned. This begins 2 cm proximal to the joint line and is carried distally and anteriorly over Gerdy's tubercle to run parallel to the lateral border of the tibial crest

fascia is left attached to the tibia to facilitate closure. A submeniscal arthrotomy is made distal to the lateral meniscus and peripheral sutures placed to aid in retraction (Fig. 2.5). This, along with the placement of a universal distractor, allows for direct visualization of the lateral joint surface. To place the distractor, one 5 mm pin is placed in the distal femur and a second 5 mm pin in the distal third of the tibial shaft where it will not interfere with the plate placement (Fig. 2.6). Any tears in the lateral meniscus can be repaired prior to closure. A Freer elevator can be used to judge the reduction of the medial aspect of the lateral plateau.

Options for Reduction and Bone Grafting

The depressed fragments of bone can be displaced far into the metaphysis of the tibia. There are a number of options to reduce these fragments. Since there is no split in the lateral cortex, as with Schatzker II fractures, direct access and elevation is not an option. The first step is to gain access to the articular fragments. A cortical window can be made in the anterolateral aspect of the metaphysis by drilling four holes with a 2.5 mm drill in a square or rectangular

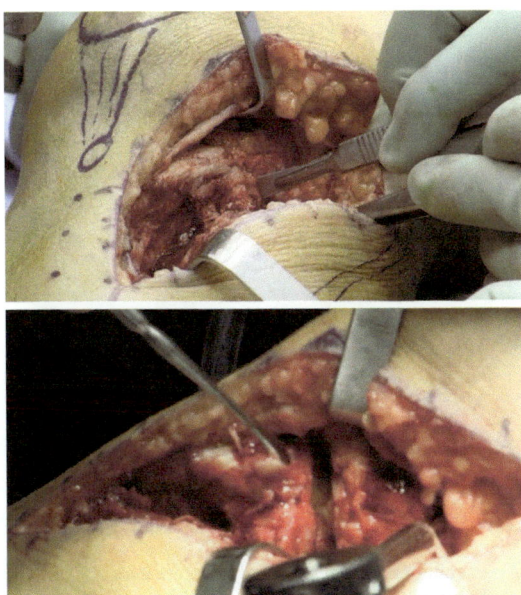

Fig. 2.5 A submeniscal arthrotomy is made to allow for direct visualization of the joint surface. Freer's elevator is helpful in palpating the fragments as they are reduced

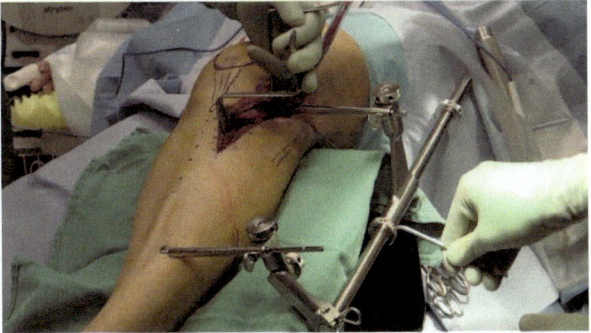

Fig. 2.6 A femoral distractor can be placed to gain length and open the lateral aspect of the knee joint. The distractor is placed such that it does not obstruct direct visualization or fluoroscopy

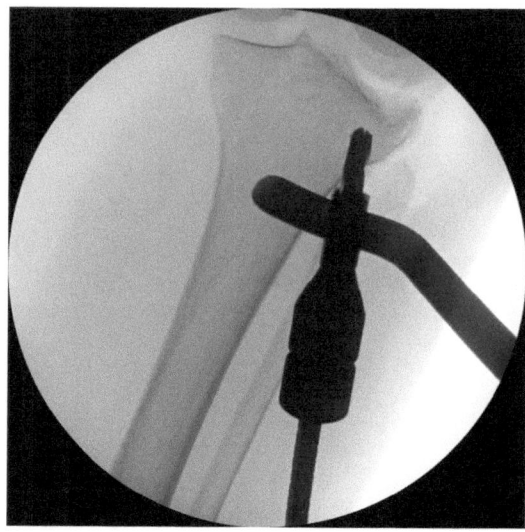

Fig. 2.7 An opening reamer can be used to create a cortical window, allowing access to the depressed fragments

pattern. A 1 cm straight osteotome is then used to connect the holes and create a window in the cortical bone. Alternatively, a 12 mm cannulated reamer can be used from the DHS set to make a window in the cortex [10]. The advantage of this is that a guide pin can be directed at the depressed fragments and location confirmed with fluoroscopy to ensure that articular fragments are easily accessible (Fig. 2.7). The window must be large enough to allow for bone grafting after the reduction. Once access is gained to the metaphysis, a curved bone tamp is then directed proximally and used to reduce the joint surface (Fig. 2.8). This is best done with light taps on the mallet rather than pushing by hand, which will allow for fine adjustments to be made to prevent joint penetration or overreduction of the fragments. The reduction can be done under fluoroscopic guidance or direct visualization through arthrotomy. Multiple passes may be required depending on the number of articular fragments and their location within the metaphysis.

Once the articular surface is restored, multiple 0.062 inch K-wires are placed under the joint surface to maintain the reduction

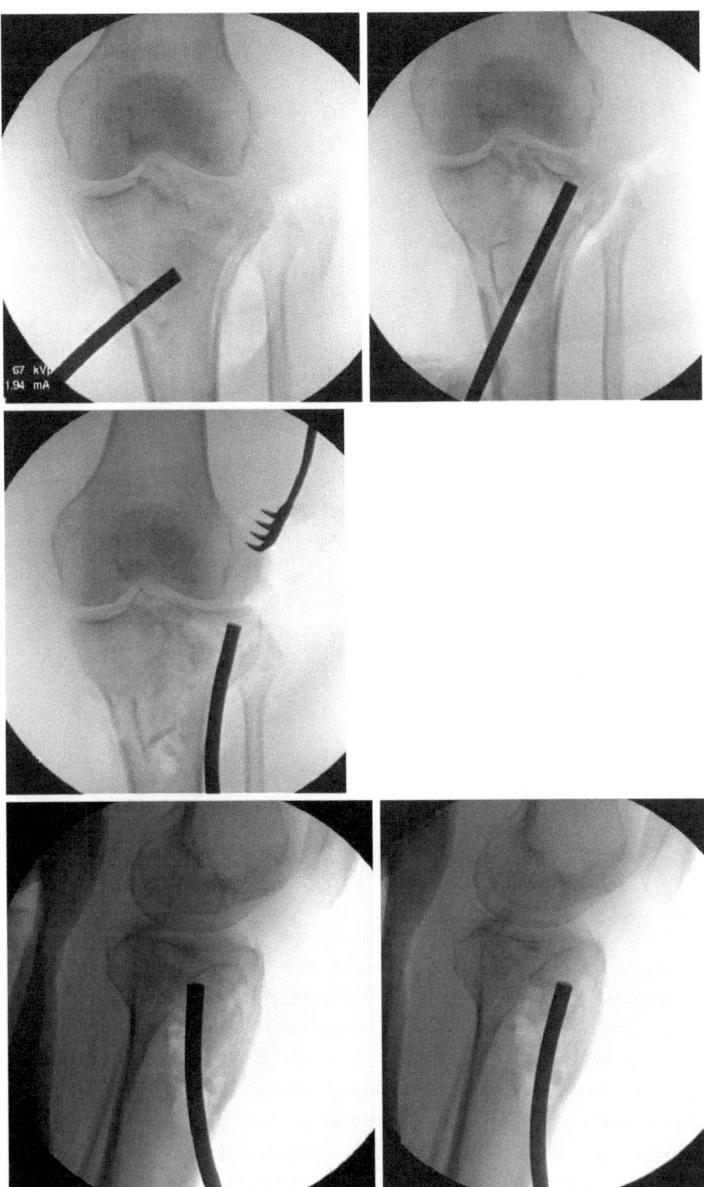

Fig. 2.8 Curved bone tamps are used to elevate the depressed articular surface under flouroscopic guidance

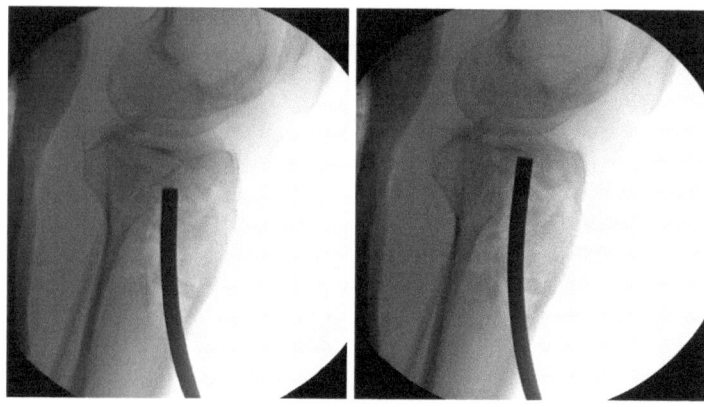

Fig. 2.8 (continued)

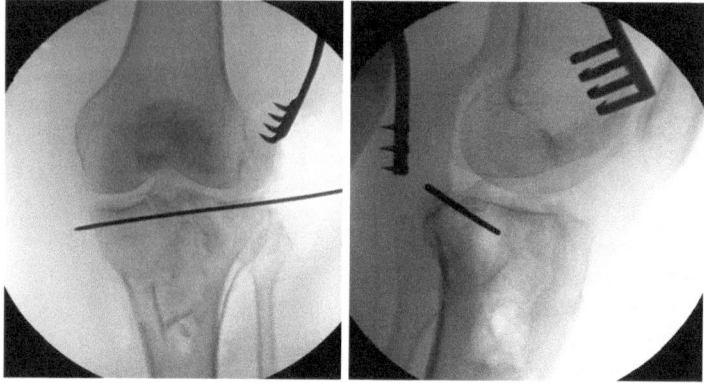

Fig. 2.9 K-wires supporting reduction

(Fig. 2.9). The joint surface is then supported with a bone graft or bone graft substitute. Allograft cancellous bone cubes provide structural support. It can be impacted under the articular surface prior to placement of definitive fixation. There is increasing evidence to support the use of biologic cements for this purpose. A number of clinical and biomechanical trials have confirmed the safety and potential benefits of using injectable calcium phosphate cement for filling bone defects [11–15]. McDonald et al. showed that calcium phosphate augmented repairs have a significantly higher fatigue strength and ultimate load compared to autografts in a cadaver model [16]. Trenholm reported less subsidence after ORIF after augmenting the reduction with calcium phosphate cement [14].

Options for Fixation

Fixation options range from percutaneously placed cannulated screws to precontoured periarticular locking plates [17, 18]. The choice of the implant is based on many factors, including the quality of bone and comminution of the fragments. The authors prefer to use a precontoured 3.5 mm nonlocking plate. The advantage of this construct is that it provides for a raft of small-diameter screws to be placed directly under the articular surface to support the reduction and prevent articular surface subsidence. A locking plate may provide more resistance to axial forces in patients with osteoporotic bone.

Newer Techniques

Recently, there have been a number of studies showing elevation of depressed bone fragments with the use of percutaneously placed, balloon-guided inflation osteoplasty [19–21]. This procedure does not require as large a cortical window in the metaphysis. A trocar for the balloon tamp is placed under fluoroscopic guidance, 2–3 mm inferior to the depressed joint surface (Fig. 2.10). A second trocar or rafting K-wires can be placed under the first trocar to direct the inflation force proximally into the depressed segments. The balloon is then inflated under fluoroscopic guidance in a stepwise fashion. The metaphyseal void is then filled with an injectable bone graft substitute (Fig. 2.11). Fixation options are the same as that for traditional methods of joint reduction. Early clinical results with this technique are promising. A number of studies show improved reductions as well as superior biomechanical properties with this technique [22].

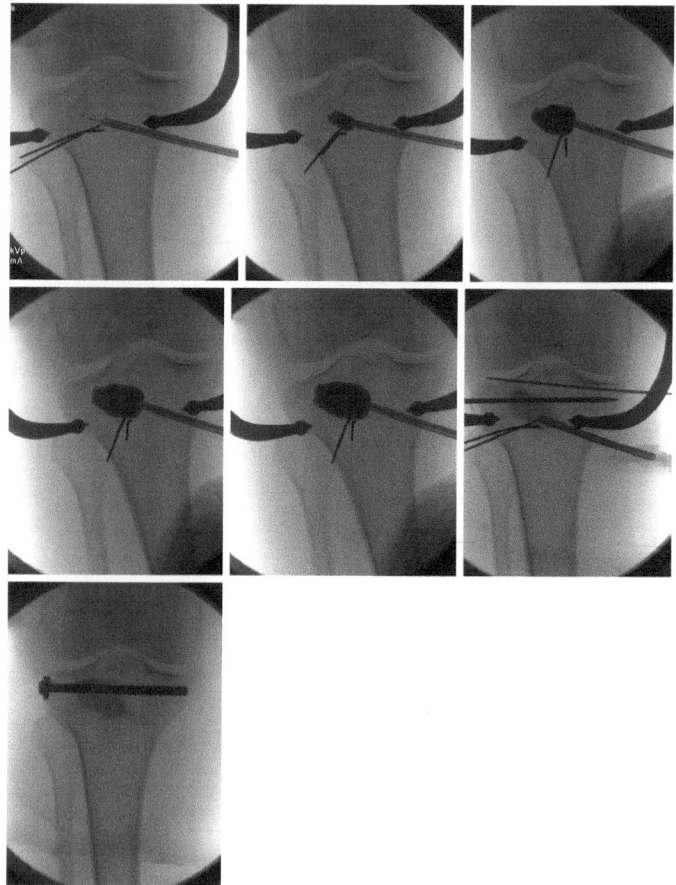

Fig. 2.10 Intraoperative fluoroscopy images demonstrating elevation of articular fragments using an inflatable balloon. Calcium phosphate is then injected, followed by percutaneous screw fixation

Postoperative Protocols Including Splint/Cast and Timing of Weight-Bearing

Postoperatively, patients are commonly placed in a hinged knee brace for 6 weeks and allowed free range of motion. Touchdown weight-bearing is recommended for the first 8–12 weeks and then advanced based on clinical and radiological evidence of fracture healing.

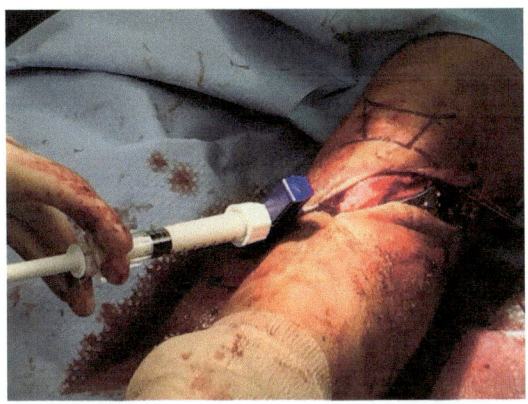

Fig. 2.11 Calcium phosphate cement is injected to fill the defect left behind after elevation of depressed fragments

Follow-Up with Union/Complications

Our patient went on to union at 17 weeks (Fig. 2.12). Her motion at last f/u was 0–120°. Overall, she was happy with her result, and she returned to her baseline activity level after 6 months.

Clinical Pearls

- Fractures of the tibial plateau with articular depression are best diagnosed and assessed with CT scan for location and degree of depression.
- Use of a bony window in the absence of a split fracture is useful to allow tamping up of the articular surface.
- Use of a guidewire from the DHS or any other cannulated system may be helpful in directing the bone tamp.
- Calcium phosphate has a higher compressive strength and ultimate load, and has been shown to decrease the articular settling after surgery, and may even allow for earlier weight-bearing.
- Use of an inflatable tamp (similar to kyphoplasty) and injecting calcium phosphate is a viable alternative for percutaneous reduction of depressed articular surface.

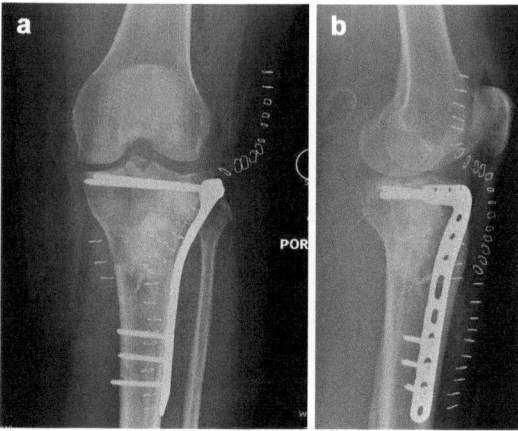

Fig. 2.12 Anteroposterior (**a**) and lateral (**b**) radiographs of the left knee demonstrating reduction of the depressed fragments with placement of a 3.5 mm periarticular locking plate. Calcium phosphate cement is seen within the metaphysis

References

1. Honkonen SE. Indications for surgical treatment of tibial condyle fractures. Clin Orthop Relat Res. 1994;302:199–205.
2. Cole P, Levy B, Watson JT, Schatzker J. Tibial plateau fractures. In: Browner BD, editor. Skeletal trauma: basic science, management, and reconstruction. Philadelphia: Saunders/Elsevier; 2009. p. 2201–87.
3. Marsh JL, Buckwalter J, Gelberman R, et al. Articular fractures: does an anatomic reduction really change the result? J Bone Joint Surg Am. 2002;84A:1259–71.
4. Giannoudis PV, Tzioupis C, Papathanassopoulos A, Obakponovwe O, Roberts C. Articular step-off and risk of post-traumatic osteoarthritis. Evidence today. Injury. 2010;41(10):986–95.
5. Macarini L, Murrone M, Marini S, et al. Tibial plateau fractures: evaluation with multidetector- CT. Radiol Med. 2004;108:503–14.
6. Chan PS, Klimkiewicz JJ, Luchetti WT, et al. Impact of CT scan on treatment plan and fracture classification of tibial plateau fractures. J Orthop Trauma. 1997;11:484–9.
7. Shepherd L, Abdollahi K, Lee J, et al. The prevalence of soft tissue injuries in nonoperative tibial plateau fractures as determined by magnetic resonance imaging. J Orthop Trauma. 2002;16:628–31.

8. Gardner MJ, Yacoubian S, Geller D, et al. The incidence of soft tissue injury in operative tibial plateau fractures: a magnetic resonance imaging analysis of 103 patients. J Orthop Trauma. 2005;19:79–84.

9. Egol KA, Tejwani NC, Capla EL, Wolinsky PL, Koval KJ. Staged management of high-energy proximal tibia fractures (OTA types 41): the results of a prospective, standardized protocol. J Orthop Trauma. 2005;19(7):448–55.

10. Hake ME, Goulet JA. Tibial plateau fractures. In: Flatow EL, editor. Atlas of essential orthopaedic procedures. Rosemont: American Academy of Orthopaedic Surgeons; 2013. p. 421–8.

11. Russell TA, Leighton RK, Alpha-BSM Tibial Plateau Fracture Study Group. Comparison of autogenous bone graft and endothermic calcium phosphate cement for defect augmentation in tibial plateau fractures. A multicenter, prospective, randomized study. J Bone Joint Surg Am. 2008;90(10):2057–61.

12. Lobenhoffer P, Gerich T, Witte F, Tscherne H. Use of an injectable calcium phosphate bone cement in the treatment of tibial plateau fractures: a prospective study of twenty-six cases with twenty-month mean follow-up. J Orthop Trauma. 2002;16(3):143–9.

13. Horstmann WG, Verheyen CC, Leemans R. An injectable calcium phosphate cement as a bone-graft substitute in the treatment of displaced lateral tibial plateau fractures. Injury. 2003;34(2):141–4.

14. Trenholm A, Landry S, McLaughlin K, et al. Comparative fixation of tibial plateau fractures using alpha-BSM, a calcium phosphate cement, versus cancellous bone graft. J Orthop Trauma. 2005;19:698–702.

15. Welch RD, Zhang H, Bronson DG. Experimental tibial plateau fractures augmented with calcium phosphate cement or autologous bone graft. J Bone Joint Surg Am. 2003;85:222–31.

16. McDonald E, Chu T, Tufaga M, Marmor M, Singh R, Yetkinler D, Matityahu A, Buckley JM, McClellan RT. Tibial plateau fracture repairs augmented with calcium phosphate cement have higher in situ fatigue strength than those with autograft. J Orthop Trauma. 2011;25(2):90–5.

17. Koval KJ, Sanders R, Borrelli J, et al. Indirect reduction and percutaneous screw fixation of displaced tibial plateau fractures. J Orthop Trauma. 1992;6:340–6.

18. Patil S, Mahon A, Green S, et al. A biomechanical study comparing a raft of 3.5 mm cortical screws with 6.5 mm cancellous screws in depressed tibial plateau fractures. Knee. 2006;13:231–5.

19. Broome B, Mauffrey C, Statton J, Voor M, Seligson D. Inflation osteoplasty: in vitro evaluation of a new technique for reducing depressed intra-articular fractures of the tibial plateau and distal radius. J Orthop Traumatol. 2012;13(2):89–95. Epub 2012 Mar 6.

20. Hahnhaussen J, Hak DJ, Weckbach S, Heiney JP, Stahel PF. Percutaneous inflation osteoplasty for indirect reduction of depressed tibial plateau fractures. Orthopedics. 2012;35(9):768–72.

21. Pizanis A, Garcia P, Pohlemann T, Burkhardt M. Balloon tibioplasty: a useful tool for reduction of tibial plateau depression fractures. J Orthop Trauma. 2012;26(7):e88–93.
22. Heiney JP, Kursa K, Schmidt AH, Stannard JP. Reduction and stabilization of depressed articular tibial plateau fractures: comparison of inflatable and conventional bone tamps: study of a cadaver model. J Bone Joint Surg Am. 2014;96(15):1273–9.

Further Reading

Biyani A, Reddy NS, Chaudhury J, et al. The results of surgical management of displaced tibial plateau fractures in the elderly. Injury. 1995;26:291–7.
Broome B, Seligson D. Inflation osteoplasty for the reduction of depressed tibial plateau fractures: description of a new technique. Eur J Orthop Surg Traumatol. 2010;20:663–6.
Hsu CJ, Chang WN, Wong CY. Surgical treatment of tibial plateau fracture in elderly patients. Arch Orthop Trauma Surg. 2001;121:67–70.
Newman JT, Smith WR, Ziran BH, Hasenboehler EA, Stahel PF, Morgan SJ. Efficacy of composite allograft and demineralized bone matrix graft in treating tibial plateau fracture with bone loss. Orthopedics. 2008;31(7):649.
Stevens DG, Beharry R, McKee MD, et al. The long-term functional outcome of operatively treated tibial plateau fractures. J Orthop Trauma. 2001; 15:312–20.

Chapter 3
Schatzker IV Tibia Plateau Fracture Treated with Open Reduction and Internal Fixation

Anjan R. Shah and Henry Claude Sagi

Case Presentation

A 67-year-old male involved in a 35 mile/h motorcycle collision. He presented to the emergency room with right lower extremity deformity. Vascular exam demonstrated an ankle brachial index (ABI) of 0.9, and tense compartments were noted on palpation. The patient was intubated secondary to closed head injury, rendering the motor and sensory exam impossible. Skin and soft-tissue envelope were intact.

A.R. Shah, MD (✉)
Florida Orthopaedic Institute, Orthopaedic Trauma Service,
13020 Telecom Parkway, North Tampa, FL 33637, USA
e-mail: anjanrshah@gmail.com

H.C. Sagi, MD
Harborview Medical Center, University of Washington, Department of Orthopedics and Sports Medicine, 325 9th Ave, Seattle, WA 98040, USA
e-mail: claudes@uw.edu

© Springer International Publishing Switzerland 2016   27
N.C. Tejwani (ed.), *Fractures of the Tibia: A Clinical Casebook*,
DOI 10.1007/978-3-319-21774-1_3

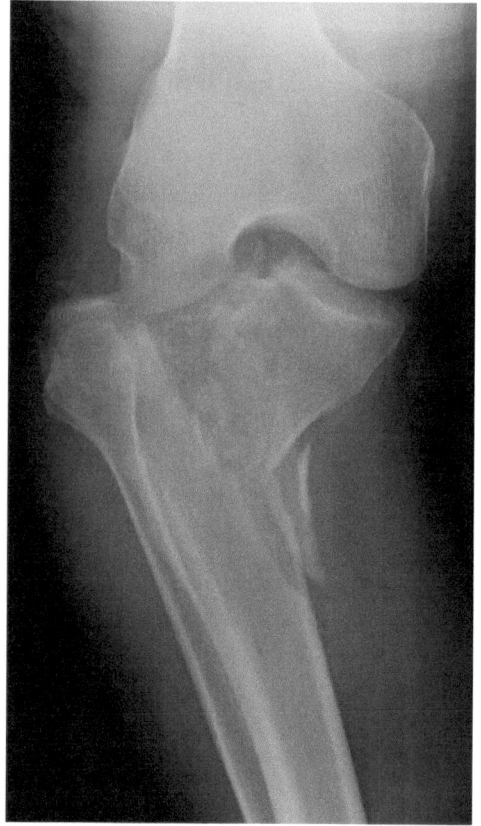

Fig. 3.1 AP Radiograph: Injury

Initial Imaging

Anteroposterior (AP) and lateral radiographs showed a displaced intraarticular medial tibial plateau fracture with dislocation of the lateral condyle (Figs. 3.1 and 3.2).

Computed tomographic (CT) scanning with angiography was performed in the trauma bay due to the abnormal ABI (Figs. 3.3, 3.4, 3.5, and 3.6).

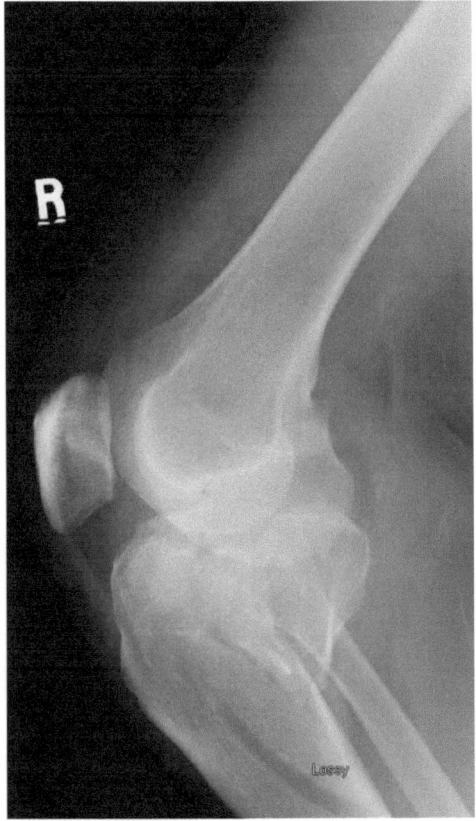

Fig. 3.2 Lateral Radiograph: Injury

Treatment and Timing of Initial Surgery

The patient was taken emergently to the operating room to undergo fasciotomies for the lower leg compartment syndrome and application of a spanning external fixator for temporary stabilization of the tibial plateau fracture. It is imperative to recognize the knee-dislocation component that can be associated with medial tibial plateau fractures, as they carry a higher

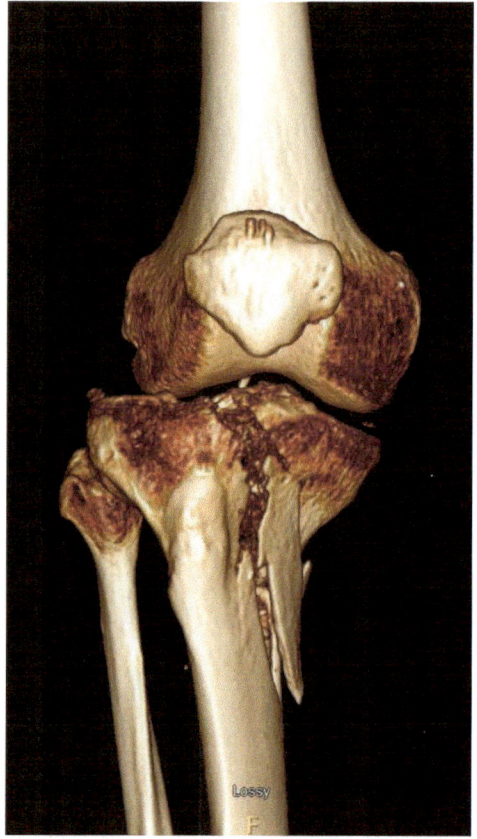

Fig. 3.3 3D Surface reconstruction CT scan: AP view, injury

incidence of neurological and vascular injuries as well as the potential for compartment syndrome.

It is the authors' preference to stage reconstruction of tibial plateau fractures associated with compartment syndrome requiring fasciotomy. Generally, the first stage involves a two-incision fasciotomy with placement of a knee-spanning external fixator to maintain length and alignment while the fasciotomy wounds heal. Because of the increased risk of infection after open reduction internal fixation (ORIF) of plateau fractures with open fasciotomy

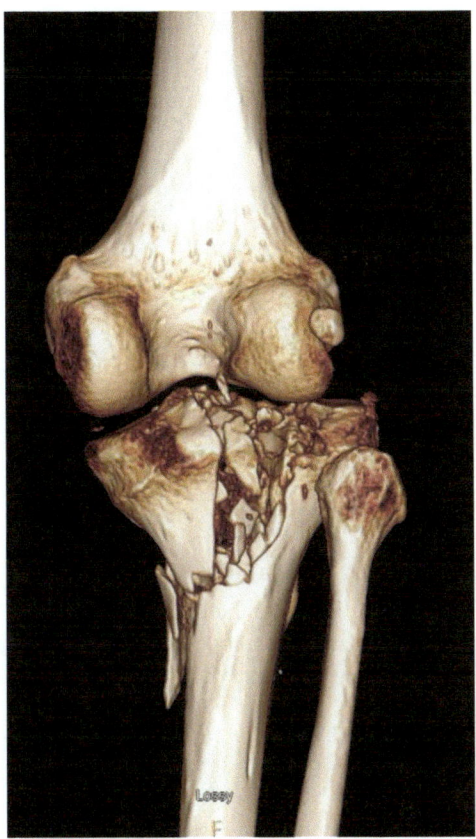

Fig. 3.4 3D Surface reconstruction CT scan: PA view, injury

wounds, definitive ORIF is not undertaken until the fasciotomy wounds are healed and free of infection (which may be anywhere from 2 to 4 weeks) (Figs. 3.7 and 3.8).

When the temporary fixator is applied, the surgeon must ensure that the lateral tibial condyle is reduced under the femoral condyle and does not remain dislocated laterally. Persistent dislocation often implies an interposed depressed osteoarticular fragment or lateral meniscus, which needs to be removed to permit reduction prior to leaving the OR (Figs. 3.9 and 3.10). If the lateral tibial condyle

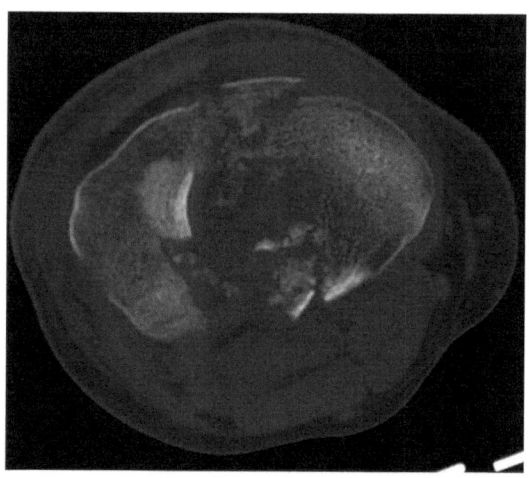

Fig. 3.5 Axial CT scan of articular surface, injury

continues to dislocate laterally, then a temporary percutaneous lag screw placed into the medial condyle can keep the lateral side from redislocating. This screw is removed at the time of definitive ORIF.

Surgical Tact

Position

Supine with bump under ipsilateral hip.

The use of a foam ramp assists in placing the knee in an appropriate amount of flexion during external fixation and also assists in radiographing imaging.

Approach

Dual-incision fasciotomies. Alternatively, a single-incision technique may be used and be particularly useful for isolated medial plateau injuries to prevent contamination of the ORIF by the fasciotomy wound. The authors place fasciotomy incisions in a man-

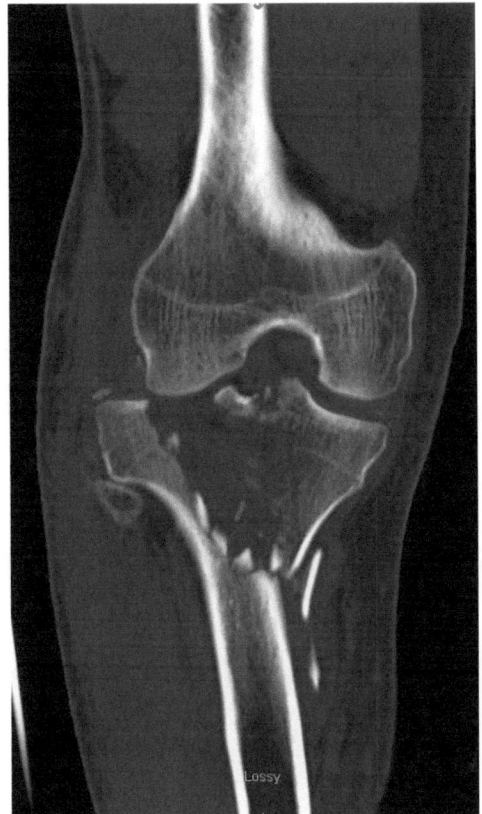

Fig. 3.6 Coronal reconstruction CT scan of injury

ner that they can be used during definitive fixation surgery, once the wounds are healed.

Pearls

- Medial tibial plateau fractures (Schatzker IV) are considered knee dislocations and hence should be evaluated for neurovascular compromise.
- The medial plateau segment in a Schatzker IV fracture acts as a constant fragment and is often well seated under the medial femoral condyle. It is the shortening and lateral translation of

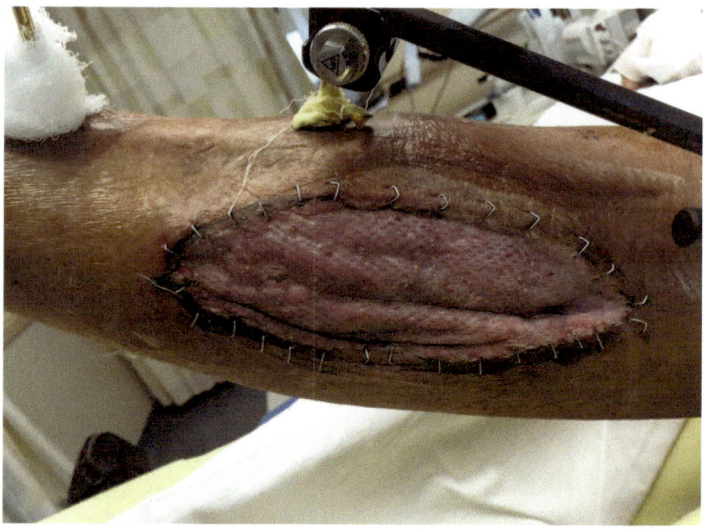

Fig. 3.7 Skin grafting of lateral fasciotomy wound

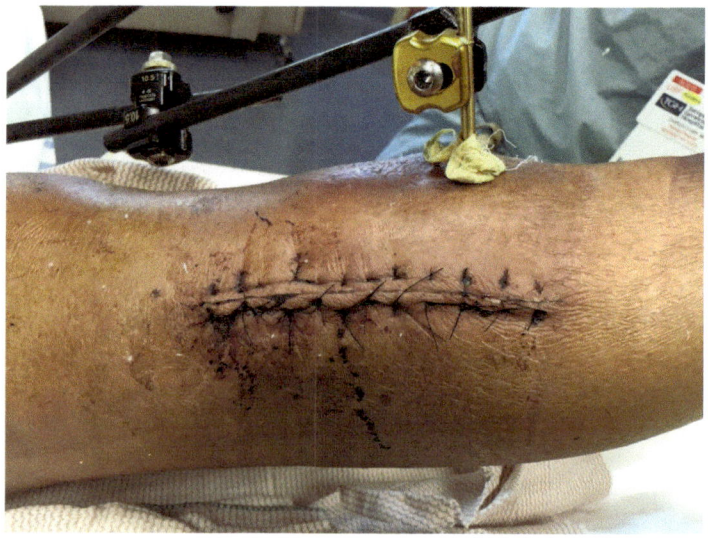

Fig. 3.8 Delayed primary closure of medial fasciotomy wound

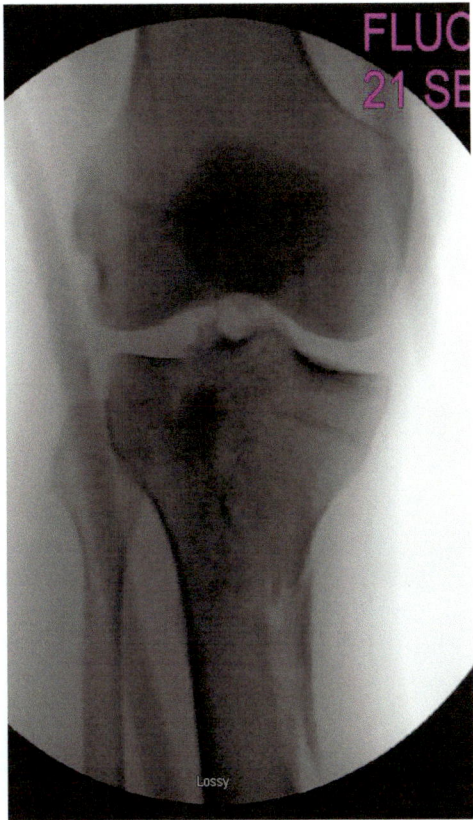

Fig. 3.9 Intraoperative AP fluoroscopic image with external fixation

the shaft and lateral plateau from beneath the lateral femoral condyle that replicate a lateral knee dislocation.

- External fixation pins should be placed well away from the zone of future definitive plate fixation and surgery to avoid contamination of the surgical site.
- Vessel loops and vacuum-assisted closure devices are utilized on the fasciotomy sites to limit skin retraction and seal the wound, limiting contamination.

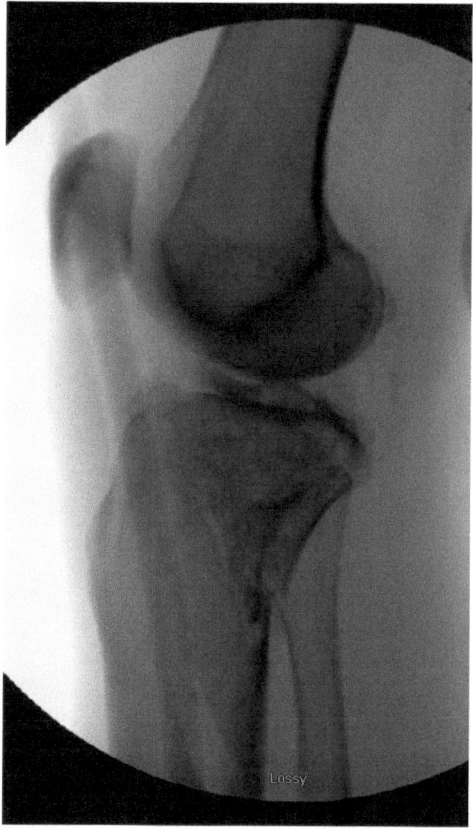

Fig. 3.10 Intraoperative lateral fluoroscopic image with external fixation

Definitive Surgery with a Posteromedial Approach

Surgical Tact

Position

The patient is positioned supine without a bump under the hip to allow for external rotation of the limb and adequate visualization of the posteromedial aspect of the affected leg.

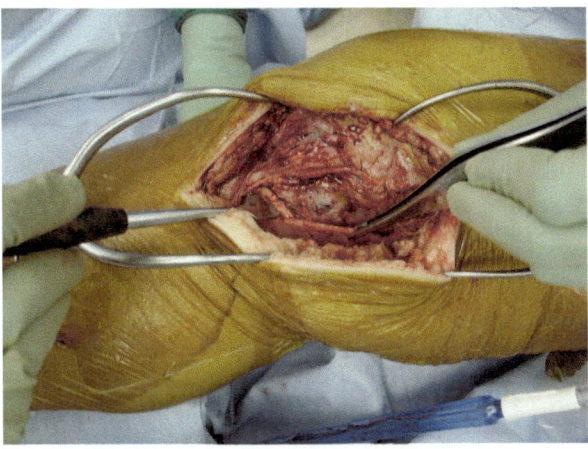

Fig. 3.11 Posteromedial exposure of pes tendons and medial collateral ligament

Surgical Approach

The incision is centered 1 cm off the posterior border of tibia and carried proximal to the knee joint by 3–4 cm. The hamstring tendons are identified and dissected to allow for mobilization; the pes anserinus insertion is preserved and retracted as needed so that the surgeon can work above and below the tendons. The superficial and deep posterior compartments are elevated subperiosteally from the posterior and medial aspect of the proximal tibia. Flexion of the knee helps to relax the gastrocnemius and popliteal neurovascular bundle, improving the surgical exposure (Fig. 3.11).

Fracture Reduction

A femoral distractor is applied to help achieve and maintain appropriate length and alignment (Figs. 3.12 and 3.13). Depressed articular segments in the medial or central aspect of the joint can be elevated using a bone tamp placed through the fracture (Fig. 3.14) and temporarily held in place with Kirschner wires. Articular fractures separating the condyles are reduced with large periarticular reduction clamps and stabilized with subchondral

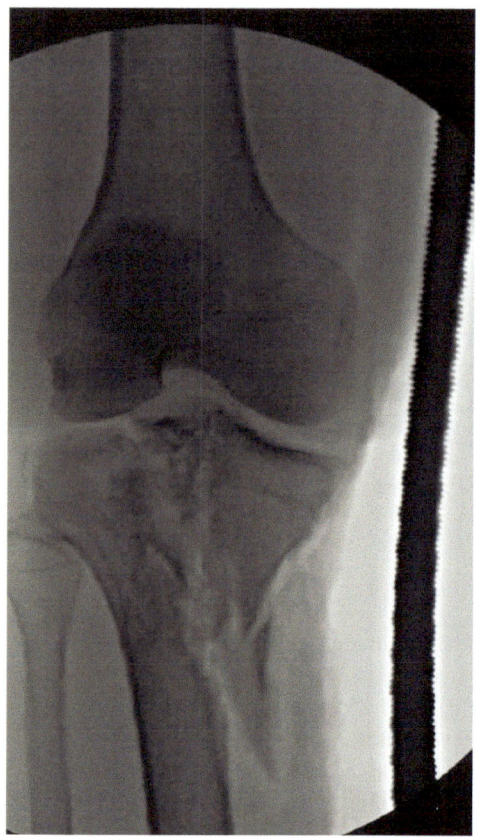

Fig. 3.12 Intraoperative AP fluoroscopic image with femoral distractor applied

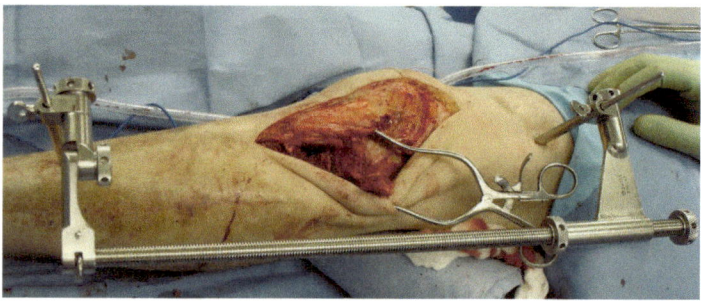

Fig. 3.13 Posteromedial exposure with universal distractor applied to regain length and aid with reduction

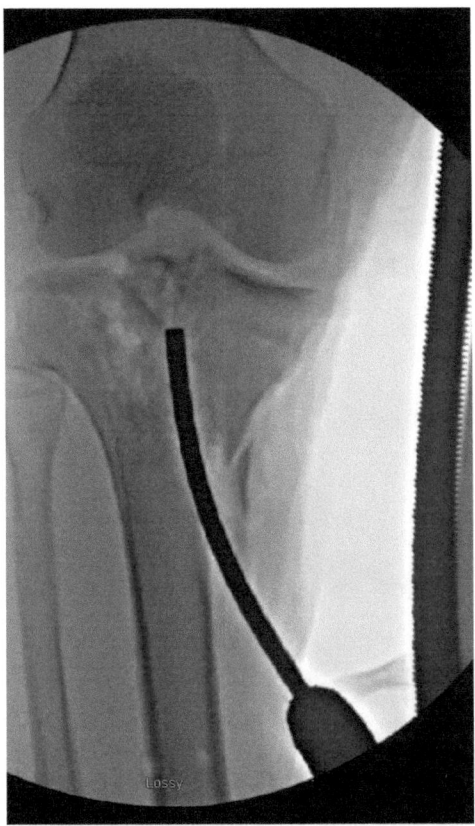

Fig. 3.14 Intraoperative AP fluoroscopic view with universal distractor applied and bone tamp through fracture to elevate depressed central articular fragment

screws of 2.7 or 3.5 mm. Coronal plane fractures that result in articular step-off can be visualized with an arthrotomy by longitudinally splitting the fibers of the deep medial collateral ligament. The fracture is compressed with a periarticular clamp and then stabilized with anterior to posterior lag screws (Figs. 3.15 and 3.16).

A posterior–medial buttress plate is applied to support the reconstruction of the posterior medial shear fragment, and the overall limb alignment and medial/lateral split is supported with a straight–medial periarticular plate (Fig. 3.17).

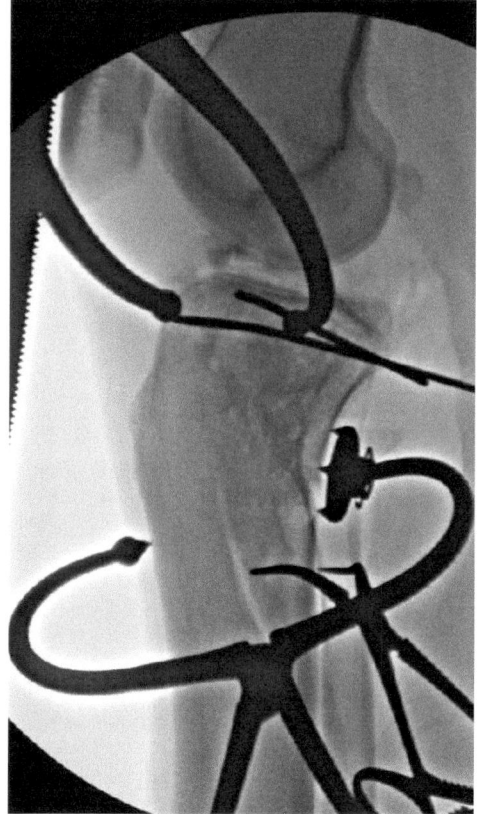

Fig. 3.15 Use of intraoperative clamps to achieve reduction

Pearls

- The spanning external fixator can be prepped into the operative field to maintain length during repair.
- Alternatively, a medially placed femoral distractor is used to restore length.
- Lighted Frazier suction tips are useful in visualization of the joint surfaces (Fig. 3.18).

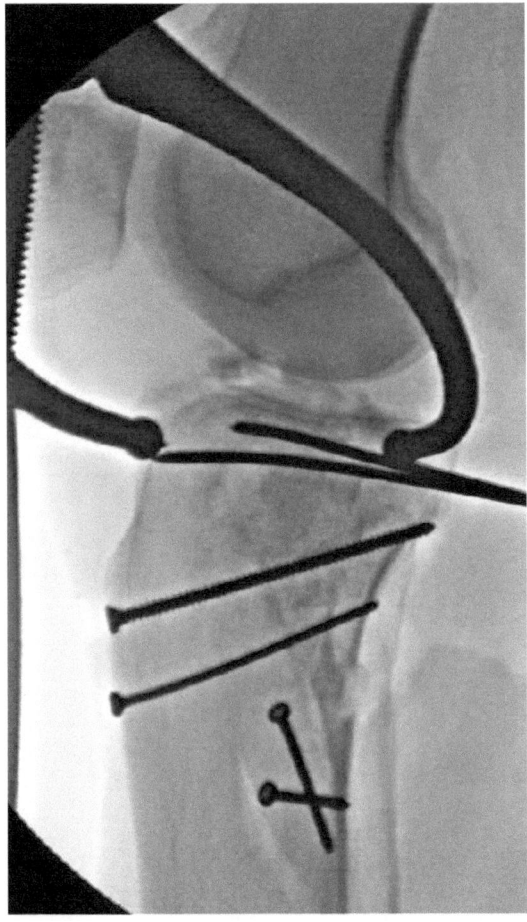

Fig. 3.16 Reduction clamps are sequentially replaced with lag or positional screws to maintain reduction

- Articular fractures should be elevated from below, maintaining a sufficient amount of subchondral bone for rafter screw support.
- Articular joint compression is paramount to achieve hyaline cartilage and not fibrocartilage formation; however, if central intraarticular comminution exists, then position screws should be placed to avoid overcompression.

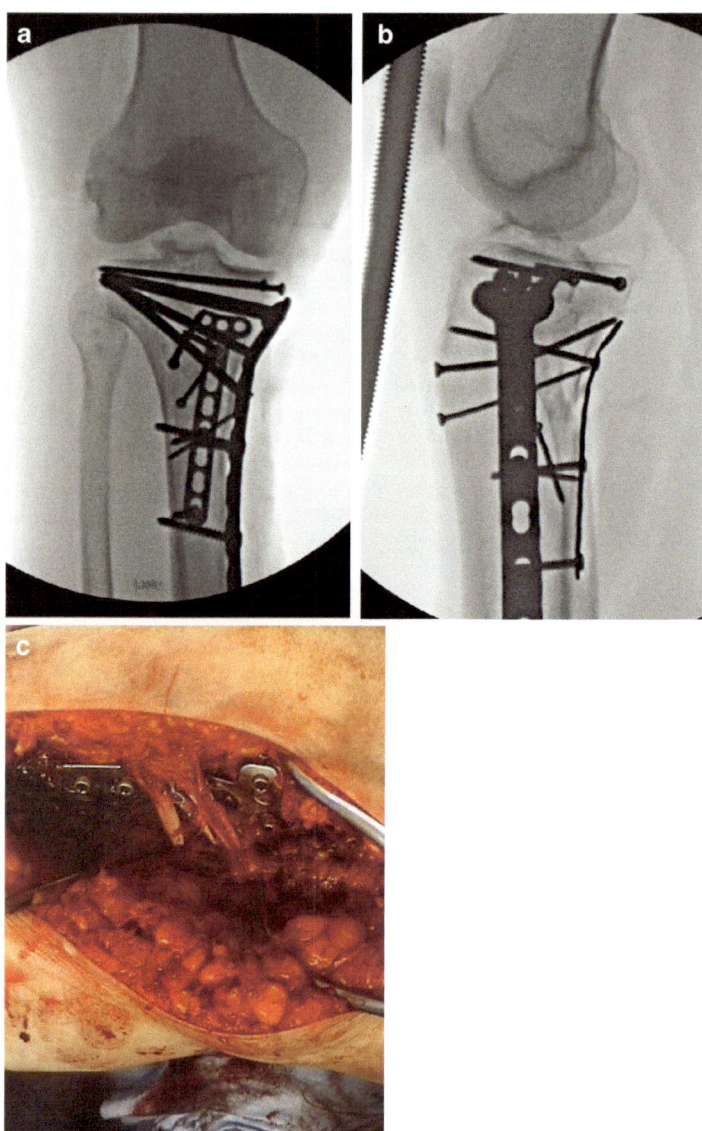

Fig. 3.17 (**a**) AP fluoroscopy showing position of posteromedial buttress plate and medial neutralization plate. (**b**) Lateral fluoroscopy. (**c**) Intraoperative picture showing plate position relative to pes tendons and MCL

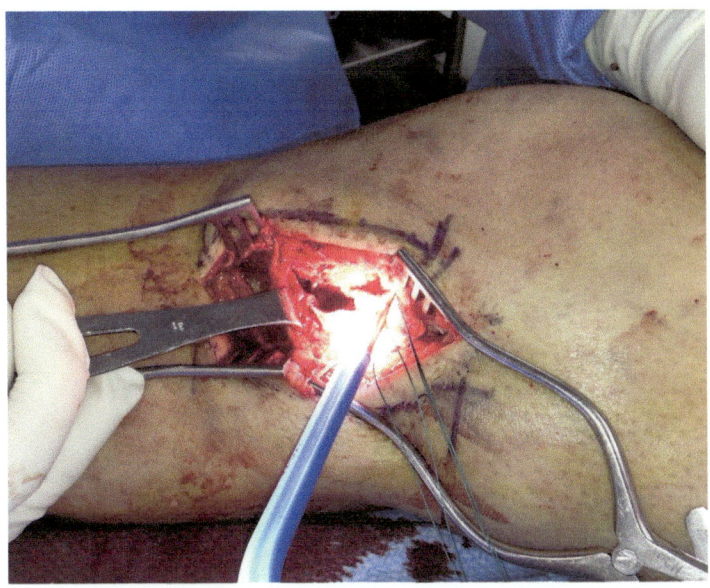

Fig. 3.18 Intraoperative lighted frazier suction tip to help with visualization of articular surface

Postoperative Plan

No knee immobilization is necessary. Immediate passive range of motion (PROM) is initiated in the postanesthetic care unit (PACU) with a continuous passive motion (CPM) machine. Full weight-bearing is permitted at 3 months (Figs. 3.15, 3.16, 3.17, and 3.18).

Chapter 4
Bicondylar Tibial Plateau ORIF Technique

Roy I. Davidovitch and David K. Galos

Introduction

Bicondylar tibial plateau fractures are complex injuries to manage. The goal, as with all fractures, is to restore length, alignment, and rotation. The two most important parameters for a good to excellent clinical outcome are restoration of the mechanical axis of the lower extremity and minimizing intraarticular incongruity [1].

Case Presentation

BB is a 29-year-old female bicyclist who was brought in by ambulance to the trauma center after being struck by a motor vehicle. She presented with an isolated injury to her left knee. Her skin was intact, and pulses were present and symmetric. She had significant swelling and effusion about the left knee. Initial imaging revealed an isolated left bicondylar tibial plateau fracture (OTA 41C3, Schatzker VI) with significant comminution and shortening (Fig. 4.1).

R.I. Davidovitch, MD (✉) • D.K. Galos, MD
Department of Orthopaedic Surgery, NYU Langone- Hospital for Joint Diseases, 301 E. 17th St., New York, NY 10003, USA
e-mail: Roy.Davidovitch@nyumc.org

© Springer International Publishing Switzerland 2016   45
N.C. Tejwani (ed.), *Fractures of the Tibia: A Clinical Casebook*,
DOI 10.1007/978-3-319-21774-1_4

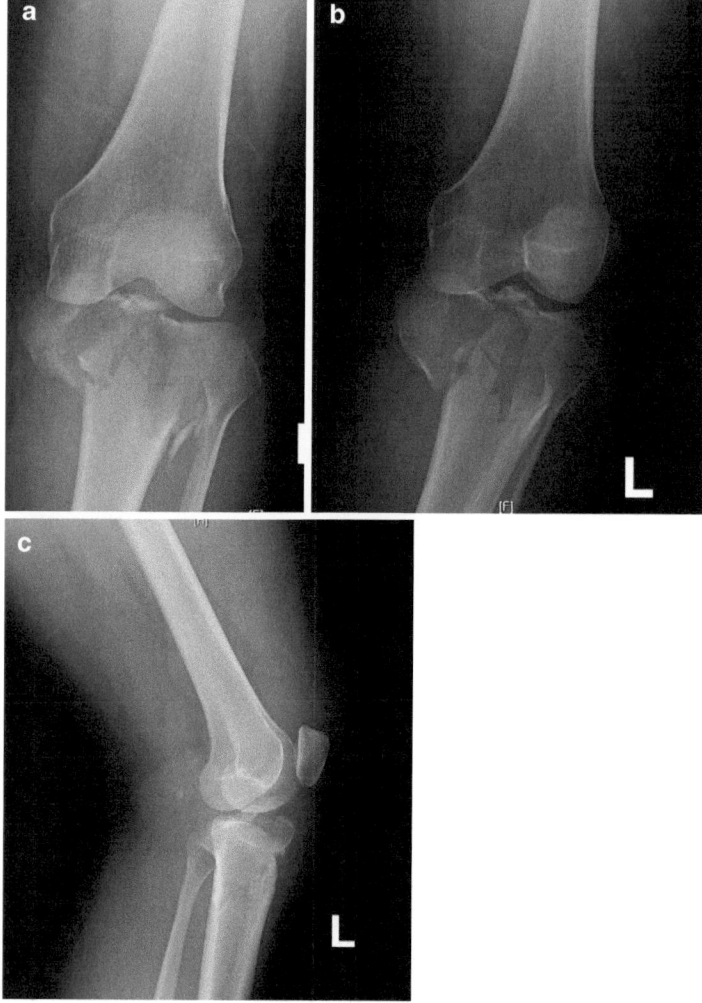

Fig. 4.1 (**a–c**) Injury radiograph demonstrating a comminuted bicondylar tibial plateau fracture

Treatment Consideration

The treatment options for bicondylar tibial plateau fractures are immediate definitive fixation, splinting, and delayed fixation after soft tissue recovery or bridging external fixation of the knee with staging to definitive fixation. Staging definitive fixation of high-energy tibial plateau fractures with spanning external fixation allows for evaluation of soft tissues, especially in patients who had open fractures and compartment syndrome, provides osseous and soft tissue stability, and helps prevent further chondral injury [2]. In addition, recent research has shown that definitive fixation of tibial plateau fractures after external fixation was not at an increased risk for infection compared to patients undergoing fixation without prior external fixation. Our indications for bridging external fixation are high-energy bicondylar fractures with significant shortening and impaction of articular surfaces and markedly swollen soft tissues that may or may not be associated with fracture blisters.

Further imaging was obtained after external fixation was placed with a computed tomography (CT) scan to better understand the fracture pattern and delineate individual fracture fragments (Fig. 4.2). CT scan has been shown to improve the interobserver and intraobserver agreement on treatment plan for tibial plateau fractures and has been shown to assist in identifying and defining posteromedial coronal fracture fragments [3]. These are important to identify, as lack of appropriate fixation into this fragment can lead to loss of reduction and overall functional outcome [4].

Computed tomography confirmed metaphyseal collapse of the medial tibial plateau with a large displaced posteromedial fragment. The lateral plateau shows no significant intraarticular depression, but there is 3–4 mm of collapse of the entire condyle. The patient was indicated for open reduction and internal fixation 18 days after injury. Our criteria for soft tissue recovery are skin wrinkling and/or decreased soft tissue edema in the area of the

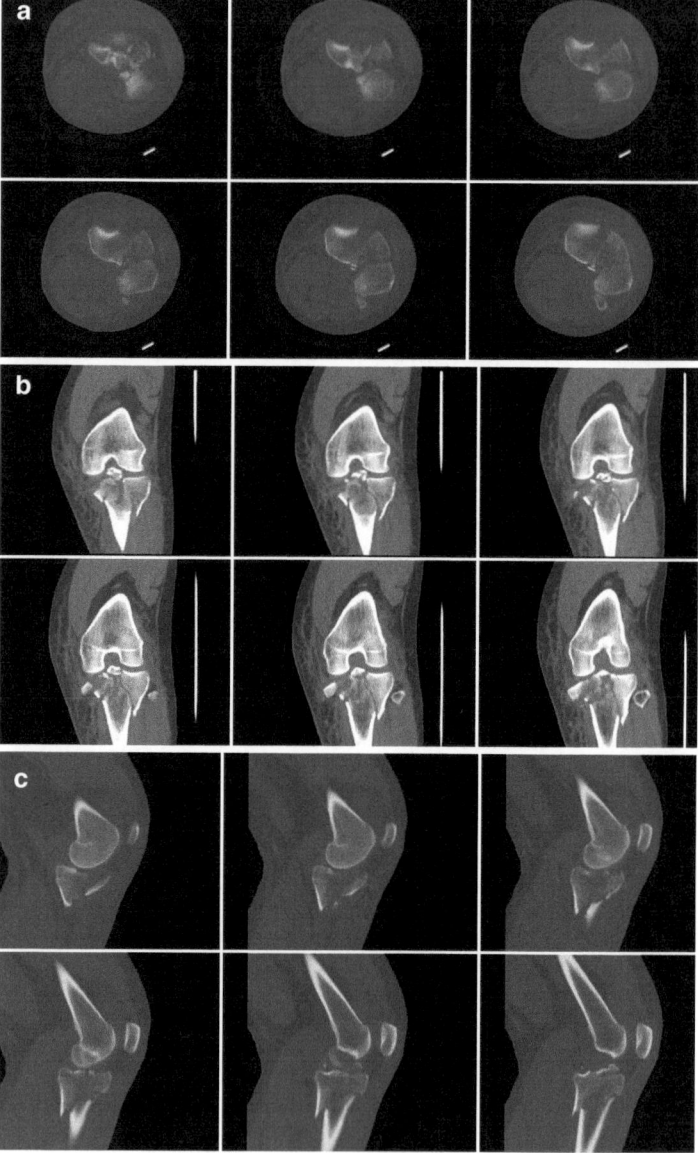

Fig. 4.2 (**a–c**) Computed tomography further demonstrating a bicondylar tibial plateau fracture, giving detailed views of each fracture fragment, amount of comminution, and joint line depression

planned incision. In instances where fracture blisters develop, we look for reepithelialization of the decompressed blisters, a process which takes roughly 7 days.

In this patient, our plan was to perform dual plating using posteromedial and anterolateral approaches. In complex, high-energy tibial plateau fractures, anterolateral and posteromedial approaches for reduction and internal fixation have been shown to improve functional outcomes and lead to acceptable radiographic reduction, especially in the presence of a posteromedial coronal split [4]. With the advent of newer locking plates, dual plating had fallen out of favor, but recent studies showed that lateral locked plating alone did not reliably secure the posteromedial plateau fragment, and that dual plating was a biomechanically superior construct [5]. The surgeon should however carefully consider dual plating approaches in patients with a high risk for wound complications, such as in diabetics and vasculopaths, as there is an increased risk for infection, which should be acknowledged [6].

Technique Details

Knee-Bridging External Fixation (Fig. 4.3)

We prefer to utilize an anteriorly based frame with the proximal pins placed through the quadriceps tendon and the distal pins anteriorly on the tibial shaft. The patient was placed in the supine position on a radiolucent table, with an image intensifier placed on the patient's right side. The extremity is placed on a bump to facilitate lateral imaging. We utilize 6 mm pins in the femur and 5 mm pins in the tibia. A simple 2 bar frame is constructed anteriorly. Fluoroscopic imaging is used to confirm that alignment is restored and that the articular surfaces are disimpacted. To make the patient more comfortable, the hematoma is usually aspirated from the joint.

Open Reduction Internal Fixation (Fig. 4.4)

The patient was placed in the supine position on a radiolucent table, with the image intensifier placed on the patient's right side.

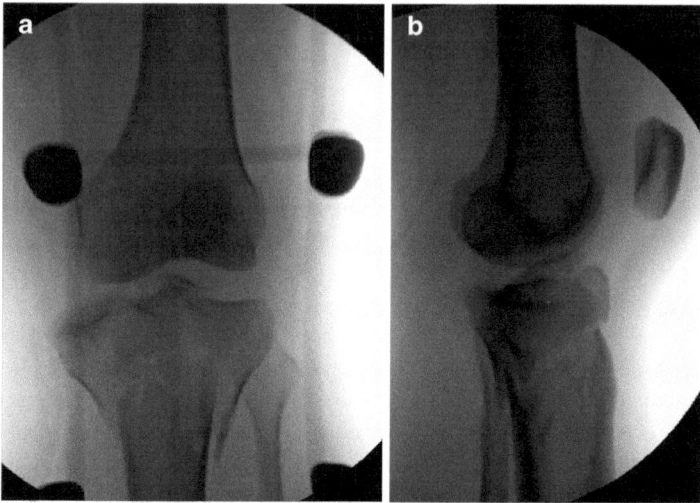

Fig. 4.3 (**a, b**) Intraoperative imaging of knee following application of external fixator

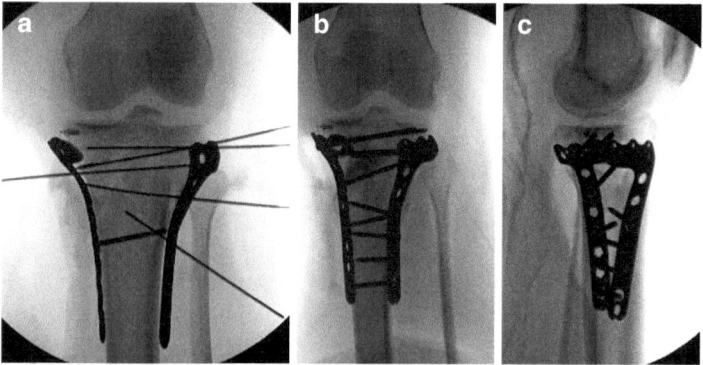

Fig. 4.4 (**a–c**) Immediate postoperative radiographs showing medial-sided antiglide plate, anterolateral precontoured plate, and a suture anchor for MCL repair. The mechanical axis and joint line appear restored and in anatomic positions

A foam bump was used to elevate the limb and allow for easy access to both the medial and lateral sides of the knee. The external fixator was removed except for a single half pin in the femur and tibia; these were prepped into the field. A tourniquet is used and inflated prior to incision to assist in visualization. A femoral distractor is then placed over the external fixation pins and is used throughout the case to facilitate intraarticular reduction.

The medial side is approached first, with a 10-cm curvilinear incision made 1 cm posterior to the posteromedial border of the tibia from 1 cm proximal to the knee. The saphenous neurovascular bundle is typically anterior to the incision however may be within the surgical field and needs to be protected. The interval between the semimembranosus and the medial head of the gastrocnemius is exploited. After skin incision is made, subcutaneous fascia is dissected until the pes anserine tendons are encountered. If necessary, the pes anserine tendon insertion may be released leaving a small tissue cuff for repair over the plate.

Once the proximal tibia is exposed, it is important to explore the integrity of the medial collateral ligament (MCL). In this particular case, the MCL was noted to be avulsed from the medial tibial plateau. This is an unusual finding in this fracture pattern. The MCL was repaired with two-suture anchors, after the plateau reduction was complete.

If significant time elapsed between injury and definitive fixation, healing may have begun, and fracture callus may be evident. This may interfere with reduction and may make attaining correct alignment with anatomic joint surface difficult. A thorough removal of the callus is necessary to allow mobilization of the facture fragments. In addition, if there is significant callus formation, the lateral side must also be mobilized prior to any reduction attempt medially. In this type of situation, the lateral incision and approach should be undertaken before any fixation is undertaken on the medial side. It is important to note that the posteromedial approach does not reliably allow for intraarticular visualization. Therefore, indirect reduction techniques relying on the reduction of the metaphyseal cortex are used to ensure that the plateau is elevated. Fluoroscopic imaging is important in judging for medial plateau reductions. Typically, the medial plateau is not comminuted, and consists of a large fragment that can be manipulated and reduced using these indirect techniques. The fracture pattern is usually a shear-type fracture; therefore, a plate in an antiglide position is the implant of choice.

In this particular case, we utilized a commercially available precontoured proximal medial tibia locking plate. The plate is slightly undercontoured to the proximal tibia. A cortical screw is placed in the tibial shaft immediately distal to the cortical spike. The plate is compressed to the shaft, and via the antiglide effect, the medial plateau is reduced into position (Fig. 4.4). Screws are not placed into the proximal aspect of the plate at this point as to avoid interfering with the lateral plateau reduction.

A lateral approach is then undertaken via a straight 10 cm incision, starting just proximal to the joint line and centered over the insertion of the iliotibial band (ITB) at Gerdy's tubercle. The incision is carried down to the ITB. A hockey stick shaped incision through the ITB and fascia is then made with the transverse limb at the level of the joint line, being careful to not violate the joint capsule, and the longitudinal limb just lateral to the tibial crest. A full thickness flap is then created, and the anterior compartment musculature is elevated in a subperiosteal fashion. A submeniscal arthrotomy was then performed, and the meniscus was freed from the fracture site. Three simple sutures were then placed through the lateral meniscus in the anterior, lateral, and posterior aspects, and small mosquito clamps were used to secure them and assist with traction proximally to allow for intraarticular visualization.

Once the fracture fragments are visualized, intraarticular and cortical callus and hematoma are removed, and fracture fragments are mobilized both medially and laterally. Once complete, the joint line is elevated in sequence from medial to lateral. K-wires of 1.25 mm are utilized to secure the fragments from lateral to medial. The K-wires are drilled flush with each fragment from lateral to medial and advanced through the skin or medial incision. This allows sequential reduction of fragments without intervening the K-wires on the lateral side. As the lateral cortical fragment is reduced, the K-wires are again drilled flush to the cortex, so that there is no interference from the K-wires when placing the plate on the lateral side.

A precontoured proximal lateral tibia locking plate of the appropriate size to allow for at least three cortical screws distal to the fracture site was chosen. The sutures from the lateral meniscus were passed through the most proximal holes and secured with mosquito clamps again, prior to securing the plate to the bone. Calcium phosphate cement was then injected through the medial fracture into the bone void left after reduction was obtained.

Final radiographs are obtained to confirm anatomic reduction and appropriate hardware placement. Special attention is paid to confirming that the joint space is not violated by any of the screws. Finally, the lateral meniscus is secured to the plate by tying the vicryl sutures down. The knee is taken through a gentle range of motion, and ligamentous stability is assessed.

A nonadherent gauze (Xeroform or Adaptec) is placed directly over the incision site, followed by gauze, loosely wrapped cotton wrap, and a loosely wrapped elastic bandage from the foot to the hip. The limb is then placed into a knee immobilizer for the patient's comfort.

Postoperative Protocol

The patient received 24 h of perioperative antibiotics with a first generation cephalosporin. Twelve hours after surgery, they were started on deep venous thrombosis (DVT) prophylaxis, which they are discharged with for 1 month.

The patient is nonweight-bearing for 12 weeks, but begin to mobilize within a hinged knee brace that is unlocked after post-op day 14. A hinged brace is discontinued after 6 weeks. The patient is discharged home once their pain is under control and they are safe to maneuver with crutches or a walker.

Our patient had no wound complications and healed well. The patient is next seen 6 weeks post-op for new radiographs to assess for healing and loss of reduction. Range of motion is assessed and should be significantly better than that at their first postoperative visit. Our patient had appropriate healing with no evidence of loss of reduction. Physical therapy is started for range-of-motion exercises of the knee, if lacking.

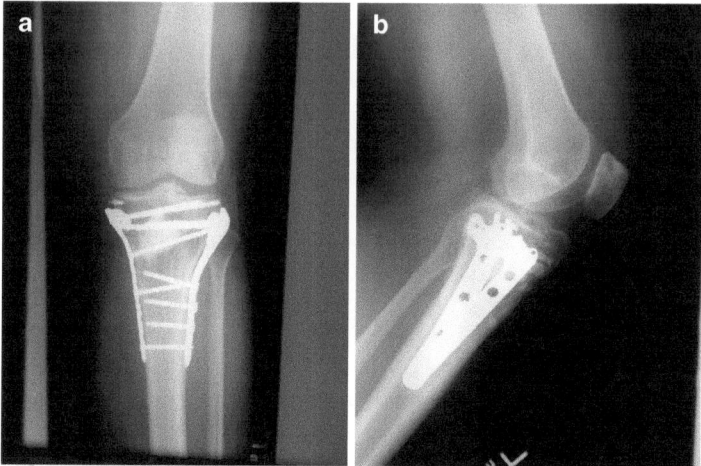

Fig. 4.5 Six-month postoperative radiographs demonstrating healed fracture with no loss of reduction

The patient is next seen at 12 weeks, and weight-bearing is advanced to as tolerated. The goal of physical therapy is to increase quadriceps strength and assist in gait training. Our patient advanced her weight-bearing and started gait training and quadriceps strengthening once full range of motion was achieved. Once full quadriceps strength was achieved, she was weaned from her assistive devices.

At our patient's next follow-up at 6 months, radiographs were obtained which showed union of her fracture (Fig. 4.5). She walked with a nonantalgic gait and had full range of motion of her knee. She was advanced to light jogging and exercises under physical therapist's supervision.

Salient Points/Pearls

- For length-unstable or widely displaced fractures, especially if there are skin issues related to blistering, a spanning external fixator is an excellent method for temporary stabilization and maintenance of length, alignment, and rotation, while the soft tissue injury resolves.

- Staged open reduction and internal fixation 1–3 weeks later has been shown to have superior outcomes as compared with acute treatment. It is important to allow for the skin to show evidence of wrinkling, which is indicative of reduced swelling.
- Typically, the medial or posteromedial fragment is initially reduced; it typically is not comminuted and has a reliable key for reduction. The lateral side is typically impacted and is approached best by direct visualization through a submeniscal arthrotomy and elevation using an osteotome.
- A bone void filler with cancellous autograft or injectable calcium phosphate may be necessary, especially if significant depression is found.
- Postoperatively, the patient should be made non-weight-bearing for a period of 10–12 weeks with early range of motion exercises in a hinged knee brace.

References

1. Giannoudis PV, Tzioupis C, Papathanassopoulos A, et al. Articular step-off and risk of post-traumatic osteoarthritis. Evidence today. Injury. 2010;41(10):986–95.
2. Egol KA, Tejwani NC, Capla EL, et al. Staged management of high-energy proximal tibia fractures (OTA types 41): the results of a prospective. J Orthop Trauma. 2005;19(7):448–55.
3. Chan PS, Klimkiewicz JJ, Luchetti WT, et al. Impact of CT scan on treatment plan and fracture classification of tibial plateau fractures. J Orthop Trauma. 2014;11(7):484–9.
4. Barei DPD, O'Mara TJT, Taitsman LAL, et al. Frequency and fracture morphology of the posteromedial fragment in bicondylar tibial plateau fracture patterns. J Orthop Trauma. 2008;22(3):176–82.
5. Yoo BJ, Beingessner DM, Barei DP. Stabilization of the posteromedial fragment in bicondylar tibial plateau fractures: a mechanical comparison of locking and nonlocking single and dual plating methods. J Trauma. 2010;69(1):148–55.
6. Barei DP. Functional outcomes of severe bicondylar tibial plateau fractures treated with dual incisions and medial and lateral plates. J Bone Joint Surg Am. 2006;88(8):1713.

Chapter 5
Bicondylar Tibial Plateau Fracture (Schatzker VI)

Kenneth Egol and John Buza

Case: Clinical History

A 59-year-old Asian American female was brought in by ambulance to the emergency department after falling down 15 steps while walking into the subway. There was no head trauma, and the Glasgow Coma Scale was 15 upon arrival. The patient's only complaint upon arrival was right knee pain. On exam, diffuse swelling and ecchymosis were noted about the right knee. The rest of the secondary exam was negative. The patient was noted to be neurovascularly intact with strong distal pulses appreciated in the right lower extremity. Radiographs were taken of the right lower extremity, as shown in Fig. 5.1a–c. The patient denied any significant past medical history. She was a retired schoolteacher, and did not smoke cigarettes or drink alcohol.

K. Egol, MD (✉)
Chief of Division of Trauma Service, Department of Orthopaedic Surgery,
Hospital for Joint Diseases, NYU Langone Medical Center, New York,
NY, USA
e-mail: Kenneth.Egol@nyumc.org

J. Buza, MD
Department of Orthopaedic Surgery,
Hospital for Joint Diseases, NYU Langone Medical Center,
New York, NY, USA

© Springer International Publishing Switzerland 2016   57
N.C. Tejwani (ed.), *Fractures of the Tibia: A Clinical Casebook*,
DOI 10.1007/978-3-319-21774-1_5

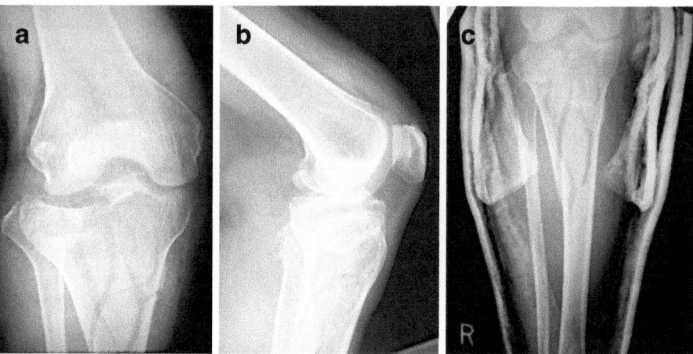

Fig. 5.1 (**a**) AP radiograph of the right knee demonstrates a bicondylar tibial plateau fracture with depression of both the medial and lateral plateaus. (**b**) Lateral radiograph of the knee further demonstrates extension of fracture into metaphysis. (**c**) AP view of the tibia demonstrates that metaphyseal comminution extends into the diaphysis, suggesting complete separation of the articular surface from the diaphysis

Diagnostic Testing and Treatment Considerations

With any suspected injury to the proximal tibia, a careful history and physical examination such as the one provided is crucial to understanding the scope and severity of injury. Identifying soft tissue injury is of paramount importance in the treatment of these injuries, as the cartilage, menisci, ligaments, and vulnerable skin envelope are all at risk. Obtaining a thorough history will provide clues to the mechanism of injury. High-energy mechanisms may be suggestive of more extensive soft tissue injury and may alter the initial workup, surgical approach, and timing of definitive treatment. In addition to the mechanism of injury, ascertaining all medical comorbidities, including smoking history, presence of diabetes, vascular disease, and congestive heart failure will provide the surgeon insight into the patient's healing capacity and may ultimately change the treatment plan.

The advanced trauma life support (ATLS) protocol will guide resuscitation and treatment of any life-threatening injuries. Knee evaluation is part of the secondary survey, which begins with examination of any open wounds, swelling, deformity, instability, or crepitus. The physical examination for the patient with a suspected tibial plateau fracture should include palpation of the suspected injury site, examination of range of knee motion, and stability to varus and valgus stress. In addition to distal pulses, obtaining an ankle–brachial index (ABI) is mandatory in any high-energy injuries when there is concern about distal flow. If the ABI is greater than 0.9, serial clinical examination of pulses, swelling, motor function, sensation, and stretch pain is strongly advised, as tibial plateau fractures may be associated with acute compartment syndrome [1]. If the ABI is less than 0.9, a reduction maneuver may be indicated along with a consult to vascular surgery for further workup, including, possibly, an arteriogram. For tibial plateau fractures with radiographic evidence of significant displacement or comminution, knee stability testing provides no additional information in the acute setting.

On presentation to the emergency department, the patient underwent a standard preoperative radiological evaluation with a knee trauma series, including anteroposterior (AP), lateral, and plateau radiographs (Fig. 5.1a–c). For displaced tibial plateau fractures, CT scan is recommended to assess the degree of comminution and depression that may be underestimated with radiographs alone (Figs. 5.2 and 5.3) [2–6]. Several authors have reported that MRI is a useful adjunct imaging modality for tibial plateau fracture [7–10]. Many authors feel as though MRI does not provide the same bony detail as CT scan for tibial plateau fractures, and therefore it is not routinely obtained at our institution in the preoperative period. In this case, the patient was found to have a bicondylar tibial plateau fracture with complete metadiaphyseal dissociation. According to the Schatzker classification, the fracture was diagnosed as Type VI [11] (Fig. 5.4).

Timing of Surgery and Preoperative Planning

Schatzker Type VI fractures typically result in a significant amount of joint instability and fracture displacement, and unless surgery is contraindicated, this injury requires ORIF for maximal restoration

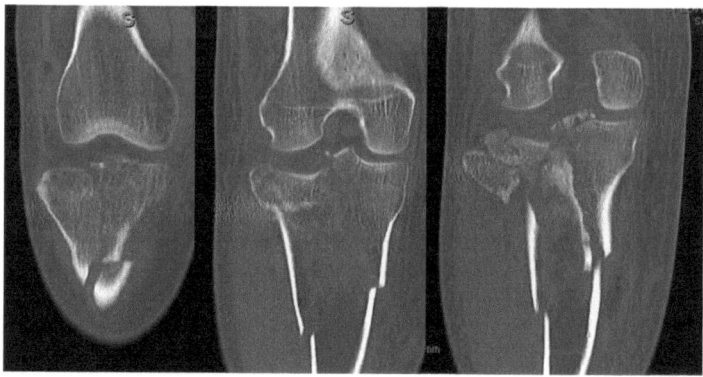

Fig. 5.2 CT reconstruction images in the coronal plane demonstrate articular impaction and comminution, particularly of the lateral condylar surface

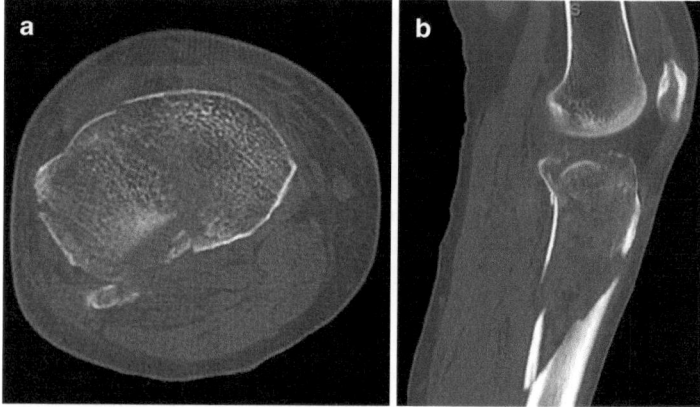

Fig. 5.3 (**a**) Axial CT cut of the articular surface demonstrating separation of medial and lateral condyles. (**b**) Sagittal CT cut further demonstrating articular impaction as well as metadiaphyseal separation

of joint congruity, axial alignment, and stability. Bracing, skeletal traction, and external fixation are all treatment alternatives, but are the exceptions to the rule, and reserved for situations in which ORIF is not possible. The timing of definitive fixation is dictated by the condition of the skin and surrounding soft tissues, which are

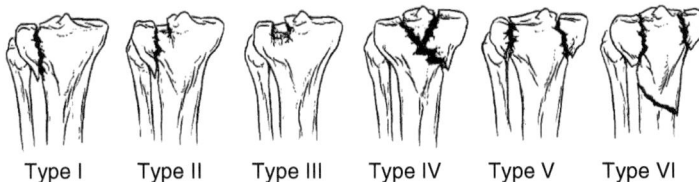

Type I   Type II   Type III   Type IV   Type V   Type VI

Fig. 5.4 The Schatzker classification of tibial plateau fractures. Schatzker Type I is a split fracture of the lateral tibial plateau. Type II is a split depression fracture of the lateral tibial plateau. Type III is a pure depression fracture of the lateral plateau without an associated split. Type IV is a fracture of the medial tibial plateau, which typically involves the entire condyle. Type V is a bicondylar fracture of both medial and lateral plateaus, usually without articular depression. Type VI is a tibial plateau fracture with an associated metadiaphyseal separation (From Koval and Helfet [29])

usually compromised in the setting of these high-energy fractures, and may be represented by open wounds, swelling, blisters, and potentially elevated compartment pressures. For all patients with a grossly unstable proximal tibia with shortening or significant soft tissue compromise, joint spanning external fixation should be strongly considered. External fixation produces stability and joint reduction through soft tissue tension, improves the quality of imaging studies, and most importantly, provides the optimal environment for soft tissue recovery and wound care (Fig. 5.5) [12, 13]. The placement of two 5–6 mm threaded half pins into the femur and tibia, with a radiolucent connecting rod and metal clamps away from the fracture zone, will accomplish all of these goals. In addition, a well-padded posterior splint will both support the leg and maintain the foot in a plantigrade position until definitive surgery. A number of clinical signs aid in determining when surgery may be safely performed: skin wrinkles, palpable bony landmarks, and the resolution of fracture blisters, extensive subcutaneous hemorrhage, or significant bruising [14].

Given the complex nature of these fractures, a thorough preoperative plan is essential to a successful outcome [15]. Surgical planning starts with careful study of the radiographs and CT scan. The surgeon must determine the location of major fracture components such as depression and splits, and plan for the use of plates and direction of screws to maintain reduction of the

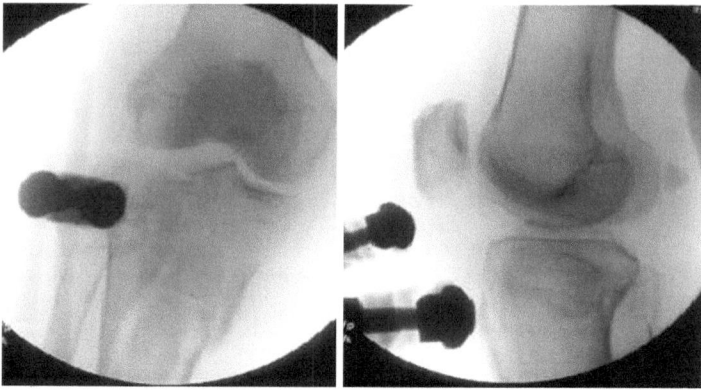

Fig. 5.5 Fluoroscopy following external fixation across the knee demonstrates improvement of the impaction at the articular surface

fragments. The surgeon may then decide which surgical approach will allow for that particular reduction and fixation. When weighing the risks and benefits of several different approaches or fixation choices, preference should be given to the soft tissues to avoid the devastating complication of wound dehiscence or skin sloughing.

Intraoperative Tips and Tricks for Reduction and Fixation

The patient should be positioned supine on a radiolucent table, with a bump under the ipsilateral hip. For posterior approaches, medial approaches, or arthroscopic-assisted procedures, positioning may vary accordingly. External fixation devices may be left in place to allow for intraoperative distraction and reduction. Placement of a tourniquet may prove useful later in the procedure, particularly during articular reduction. For fractures with significant lower extremity malalignment, including the contralateral leg in the operative leg may help with the assessment of the lower extremity alignment. A large C-arm fluoroscope should be placed on the opposite side of the operative field, and directly perpendicular to the patient. Although not necessary, placement of a femoral distractor greatly assists in visualization of the femorotibial joint. If external fixation has not been used, the distractor is applied using a single 5 mm Schanz pin across the femoral condyles, and another across the tibia, distal to the fracture site. Placement of the distractor on the lateral side of the joint allows better access to the lateral compartment, which commonly has the greater degree of comminution.

Articular reduction is accomplished by elevating any impacted articular fragments from below the joint. These articular fragments will fall back into the metaphyseal void unless supported adequately. There are a number of bone void filler options, including autograft cancellous bone graft, freeze-dried human demineralized bone matrix, calcium sulfate materials, and hydroxyapatite materials. After provisional reduction of the articular surface with K-wire fixation, raft screws are placed. This construct has been shown to prevent the loss of articular surface reduction (Fig. 5.6a, b) [16–18]. Long 3.5 mm cortical screws must capture both the

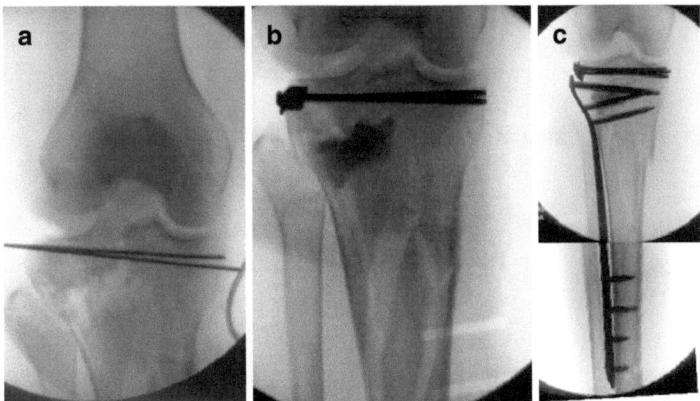

Fig. 5.6 (**a**) Provisional K-wire fixation across the elevated articular fragments temporarily maintains reduction. (**b**) Replaced with a raft screw/rim plate construct across the subchondral bone, capturing both medial and lateral cortices, acts to support the articular cartilage and prevent loss of reduction. Bone cement has been injected into the metaphyseal void caused by articular impaction. (**c**) Following articular reduction, placement of a locked plate allows further reduction of the medial plateau and metadiaphyseal fixation

plate and the far cortex, thereby transmitting force across the joint to both medial and lateral cortices [19]. These screws can be placed through specially designed precontoured plates, if possible; otherwise, they should be placed outside of the plate.

Following articular reduction, an implant must be selected, which can both prevent collapse of a fixed plateau and connect the articular surface to the diaphysis in satisfactory alignment. Unlike the articular surface, metadiaphyseal fracture healing is more amenable to relative-stability constructs such as bridge plates. A number of low-profile precontoured plates specifically designed to fit the proximal tibia are available that may serve this purpose. The advent of the angular stable locked plate has gained significant interest and use in the treatment of bicondylar tibial plateau fractures in recent years, and will be discussed further in the section below [20–23]. Despite their popularity, it is important to remember that locked plates are not a panacea; the technique is technically difficult and demanding. For example, bicolumnar fractures with poor reduction of the medial column tend to fall into varus with cyclical loading. For this reason, many surgeons prefer a dual-plate approach in which an antiglide plate can be placed at the apex of the posteromedial spike for anatomic reduction. Perhaps, the most important aspect of this technique is proper planning to allow for minimal soft tissue dissection, as a second incision increases the risk of infection and wound problems.

Technique of Open Reduction and Internal Fixation

Plates and screws are the mainstays of implants utilized for these fractures. Locked angular-stable implants are able to control bone alignment without relying on friction at the bone-implant interface, and therefore can span the entire fracture site and potentially allow for fixation of a bicondylar fracture with one implant. An anterolateral approach to the proximal tibia allows good access for placement of any lateral-based plate. Distraction, K-wires, and periarticular reduction clamps can all be used to help align major condylar fracture fragments [24]. For a lateral-based locking plate, the medial and lateral condyles are reduced first, and then reconnected to the diaphysis. Kirschner wires help to maintain the reduction temporarily. Articular impaction is then reduced through either an anterior fracture split or after creating a submetaphyseal cortical window (Fig. 5.7a). After fixation of fracture fragments with K-wires or raft screws, the lateral locking plate may be applied (Fig. 5.7b). If only a lateral locking plate is used, it is crucial that cortical contact is reestablished at the base of the medial condyle. If this cannot be achieved, then a small posteromedial incision and application of an antiglide or one-third tubular plate

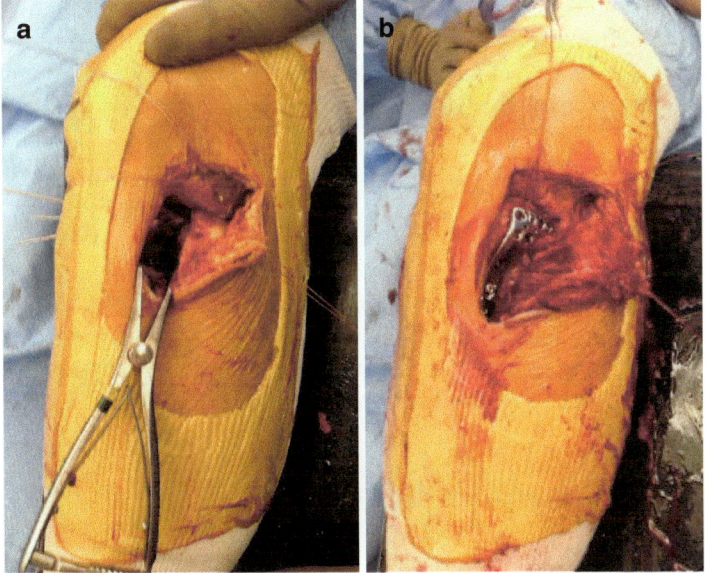

Fig. 5.7 Example of application of a lateral-based locking plate. (**a**) Reduction of any articular impaction may be achieved through an anterior fracture split. (**b**) Lateral locking plate in place following reduction of the articular surface

at the apex of the posteromedial spike may be required. Prior to fixation of the implant, it is also important to reestablish alignment of the lower extremity.

Following reduction of the articular surface and provisional fixation in acceptable anatomic alignment, the plate may be secured to the tibia. If a locked plating system is used, it is important that the surgeon be familiar with the instrumentation. Considering these plates can be placed in a submuscular fashion, the incisions may be kept smaller, which may help to preserve blood flow to the metaphyseal region. Although most screws can be inserted percutaneously, it is important to remember that the most distal screws should be placed using a 2–4 cm incision and blunt dissection to visualize the tibia, as studies have demonstrated increased risk of neurovascular damage at these positions [25]. Following surgery completion, external fixation pins, if used, should be removed, and the knee manipulated and flexed to lyse any adhesions that may have developed during the period of temporary external fixation.

Postoperative Protocol

Patients are immobilized for 7–10 days. Our protocol is to keep patients non-weight-bearing for 10 weeks, but begin early quadriceps-strengthening exercises, and then to gradually advance to full weight-bearing by 12 weeks. We prefer to institute early range of knee motion to minimize stiffness.

Follow-Up and Complications

Careful preoperative planning, close attention to the status of the soft tissues, and improved surgical techniques have all decreased the prevalence of complications in the treatment of tibial plateau fractures. Wound breakdown and infection are serious complications that may result from incisions through traumatized soft tissue [26, 27]. Should superficial breakdown occur, immediate irrigation and debridement is necessary. Deeper wound breakdown may require free flap or rotational flap closure in addition to irrigation and debridement.

Aseptic nonunion at the metadiaphyseal junction is uncommon, but can be seen following high-energy Schatzker V or VI fracture patterns [27, 28]. Again, if this develops, it should be treated early with bone grafting with possible revision of fixation. If malalignment of the lower extremity occurs in conjunction, an osteotomy may be required to correct the deformity. Articular surface malunions or posttraumatic arthritis in elderly patients may be treated with total knee arthroplasty. Close follow-up of patients following high-energy tibial plateau fractures is important to observe for both wound-healing and bone-healing complications (Figs. 5.8, 5.9, and 5.10)

Salient Points/Pearls

- Bicondylar tibial plateau fractures are high-energy injuries, and associated injuries should be looked for including compartment syndrome, neurological, and vascular injuries.

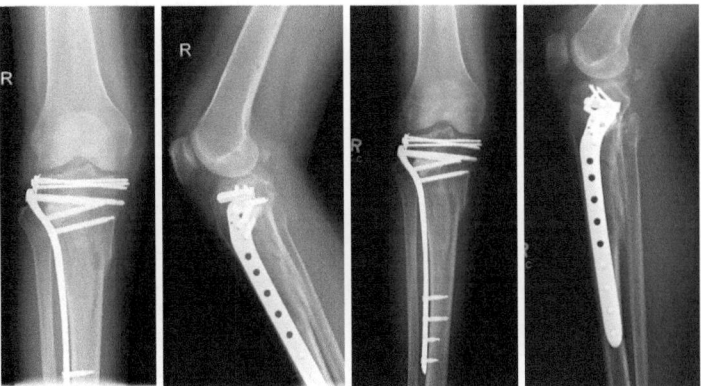

Fig. 5.8 AP and lateral radiographs of the knee and tibia/fibula taken 3 months following surgery. Radiographs demonstrate maintenance of the articular surface, good anatomic alignment, and evidence of fracture healing

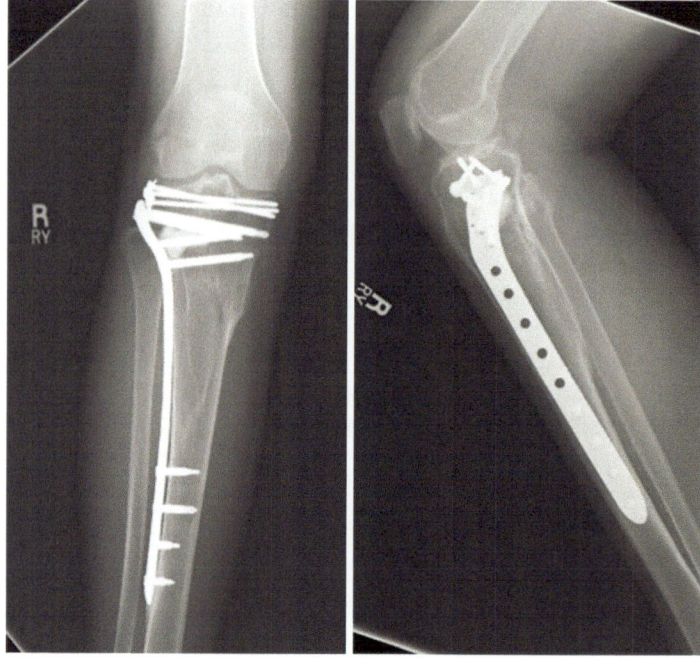

Fig. 5.9 AP and lateral radiographs of the tibia/fibula taken 1.5 years following surgery. Radiographs demonstrate maintenance of the articular surface, good anatomic alignment, and evidence of fracture healing

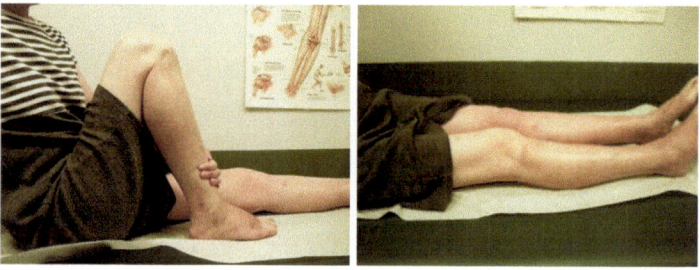

Fig. 5.10 Examination of the patient at 1.5 years following surgery reveals a range of motion of 0–130°

- Use of a spanning, temporary external fixation is useful in allowing soft tissue management and time for surgical planning.
- It may take 1–3 weeks for swelling to decrease to allow for safe surgical intervention.
- Dual plating is the preferred option with dual incisions, even with use of locking plates.
- Early range of motion will allow for improved outcomes.

References

1. Andrews JR, Tedder JL, Godbout BP. Bicondylar tibial plateau fracture complicated by compartment syndrome. Orthop Rev. 1992;21(3):317–9.
2. Rafii M, Firooznia H, Golimbu C, Bonamo J. Computed tomography of tibial plateau fractures. AJR Am J Roentgenol. 1984;142(6):1181–6.
3. Dias JJ, Stirling AJ, Finlay DB, Gregg PJ. Computerised axial tomography for tibial plateau fractures. J Bone Joint Surg. 1987;69(1):84–8.
4. Chan PS, Klimkiewicz JJ, Luchetti WT, et al. Impact of CT scan on treatment plan and fracture classification of tibial plateau fractures. J Orthop Trauma. 1997;11(7):484–9.
5. Liow RY, Birdsall PD, Mucci B, Greiss ME. Spiral computed tomography with two- and three-dimensional reconstruction in the management of tibial plateau fractures. Orthopedics. 1999;22(10):929–32.
6. Macarini L, Murrone M, Marini S, Calbi R, Solarino M, Moretti B. Tibial plateau fractures: evaluation with multidetector-CT. Radiol Med. 2004;108(5–6):503–14.
7. Kode L, Lieberman JM, Motta AO, Wilber JH, Vasen A, Yagan R. Evaluation of tibial plateau fractures: efficacy of MR imaging compared with CT. AJR Am J Roentgenol. 1994;163(1):141–7.
8. Holt MD, Williams LA, Dent CM. MRI in the management of tibial plateau fractures. Injury. 1995;26(9):595–9.
9. Yacoubian SV, Nevins RT, Sallis JG, Potter HG, Lorich DG. Impact of MRI on treatment plan and fracture classification of tibial plateau fractures. J Orthop Trauma. 2002;16(9):632–7.
10. Gardner MJ, Yacoubian S, Geller D, et al. The incidence of soft tissue injury in operative tibial plateau fractures: a magnetic resonance imaging analysis of 103 patients. J Orthop Trauma. 2005;19(2):79–84.
11. Schatzker J, McBroom R, Bruce D. The tibial plateau fracture. The Toronto experience 1968–1975. Clin Orthop Relat Res. 1979;1979(138):94–104.
12. Egol KA, Tejwani NC, Capla EL, Wolinsky PL, Koval KJ. Staged management of high-energy proximal tibia fractures (OTA types 41): the

results of a prospective, standardized protocol. J Orthop Trauma. 2005;19(7):448–55. discussion 456.

13. Laible C, Earl-Royal E, Davidovitch R, Walsh M, Egol KA. Infection after spanning external fixation for high-energy tibial plateau fractures: is pin site-plate overlap a problem? J Orthop Trauma. 2012;26(2):92–7.

14. Strauss EJ, Petrucelli G, Bong M, Koval KJ, Egol KA. Blisters associated with lower-extremity fracture: results of a prospective treatment protocol. J Orthop Trauma. 2006;20(9):618–22.

15. Egol KA, Koval KJ. Fractures of the proximal tibia. In: Buchholz RW, Heckman JD, Court-Brown CM, editors. Rockwood & green's fractures in adults, vol 6th ed. Philadelphia: Lippincott Williams and Wilkins; 2006.

16. Beris AE, Soucacos PN, Glisson RR, Seaber AV, Urbaniak JR. Load tolerance of tibial plateau depressions reinforced with a cluster of K-wires. Bull Hosp Jt Dis. 1996;55(1):12–5.

17. Karunakar MA, Egol KA, Peindl R, Harrow ME, Bosse MJ, Kellam JF. Split depression tibial plateau fractures: a biomechanical study. J Orthop Trauma. 2002;16(3):172–7.

18. Patil S, Mahon A, Green S, McMurtry I, Port A. A biomechanical study comparing a raft of 3.5 mm cortical screws with 6.5 mm cancellous screws in depressed tibial plateau fractures. Knee. 2006;13(3):231–5.

19. Cooper HJ, Kummer FJ, Egol KA, Koval KJ. The effect of screw type on the fixation of depressed fragments in tibial plateau fractures. Bull Hosp Jt Dis. 2001;60(2):72–5.

20. Ricci WM, Rudzki JR, Borrelli Jr J. Treatment of complex proximal tibia fractures with the less invasive skeletal stabilization system. J Orthop Trauma. 2004;18(8):521–7.

21. Cole PA, Zlowodzki M, Kregor PJ. Treatment of proximal tibia fractures using the less invasive stabilization system: surgical experience and early clinical results in 77 fractures. J Orthop Trauma. 2004;18(8):528–35.

22. Egol KA, Su E, Tejwani NC, Sims SH, Kummer FJ, Koval KJ. Treatment of complex tibial plateau fractures using the less invasive stabilization system plate: clinical experience and a laboratory comparison with double plating. J Trauma. 2004;57(2):340–6.

23. Bonyun M, Nauth A, Egol KA, et al. Hot topics in biomechanically directed fracture fixation. J Orthop Trauma. 2014;28 Suppl 1:S32–5.

24. Egol KA, Koval KJ. Fractures of the tibial plateau. In: Chapman MW, editor. Chapman;s orthopaedic surgery, vol 3rd ed. Philadelphia: Lippincott Williams & Wilkins; 2001.

25. Deangelis JP, Deangelis NA, Anderson R. Anatomy of the superficial peroneal nerve in relation to fixation of tibia fractures with the less invasive stabilization system. J Orthop Trauma. 2004;18(8):536–9.

26. Young MJ, Barrack RL. Complications of internal fixation of tibial plateau fractures. Orthop Rev. 1994;23(2):149–54.

27. Weiner LS, Kelley M, Yang E, et al. The use of combination internal fixation and hybrid external fixation in severe proximal tibia fractures. J Orthop Trauma. 1995;9(3):244–50.
28. Watson JT. High-energy fractures of the tibial plateau. Orthop Clin North Am. 1994;25(4):723–52.
29. Koval K, Helfet D. Tibial plateau fractures. J Am Acad Orthop Surg. 1995;3:86–94.

Chapter 6
Tibial Plateau Schatzker V/VI Treated in Ex Fix/Circular Frame

James Lachman and Saqib Rehman

History

The patient is an 18-year-old female with no past medical history other than borderline mental retardation who presents after an urban all-terrain vehicle (ATV) accident where she was thrown from the vehicle. On initial evaluation in the trauma bay, she was noted to have a 15×6 cm wound over her anteromedial leg, with significant degloving over the tibia. She was found to have a Schatzker VI tibial plateau fracture with large (Gustilo Anderson IIIB) metadiaphyseal butterfly fragment (Fig. 6.1). She also was found to have a nondisplaced medial malleolus fracture on the ipsilateral side.

J. Lachman, MD (✉) • S. Rehman, MD
Department of Orthopaedic Surgery, Temple University,
Philadelphia, PA, USA
e-mail: james.lachman2@tuhs.temple.edu

© Springer International Publishing Switzerland 2016   73
N.C. Tejwani (ed.), *Fractures of the Tibia: A Clinical Casebook*,
DOI 10.1007/978-3-319-21774-1_6

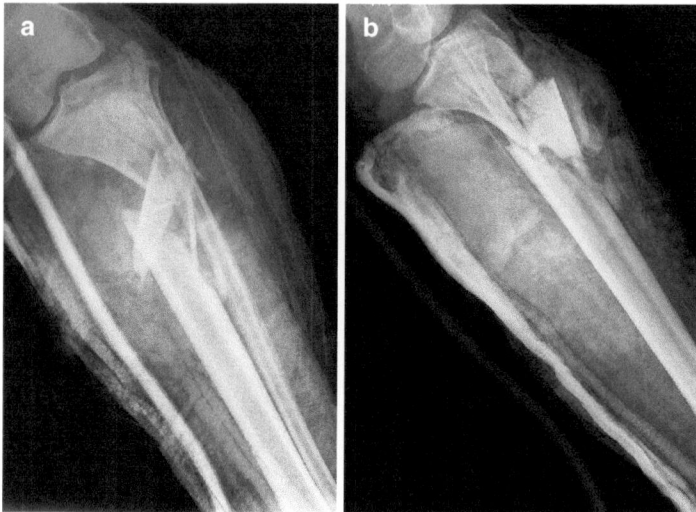

Fig. 6.1 Initial presentation. (**a, b**) Initial AP and lateral radiographs demonstrating a bicondylar tibial plateau fracture with depressed lateral condyle and metaphyseal diaphyseal comminution

Treatment Considerations/Planning/Tests Needed

The major considerations of this case are as follows:

1. There is severe soft tissue injury with skin loss. Preventing infection through thorough debridement and early and adequate soft tissue coverage is necessary.
2. The fracture involves some metaphyseal bone loss, but the articular injury and joint depression are mild to moderate. This will simplify the treatment with regard to surgical approach, in particular.
3. The patient is young, relatively healthy with no systemic disease, and is a nonsmoker, which should bode well for bony and soft tissue healing. However, there were significant concerns regarding her follow-up and aftercare. Although she was deemed mentally competent to make medical decisions, her insight into her condition was poor, and her social support was suspected to be inadequate. Open Schatzker V/VI injuries

generally require months of follow-up (or longer), with the potential for several surgeries "down the road"; so, patient compliance and expectations are important to establish early in the treatment process.

Surgical Tact

The patient was brought emergently to the operating room for irrigation and debridement of the grade IIIB open fracture with placement of antibiotic beads and negative pressure therapy-assisted closure. A large portion of her anterior tibial metadiaphysis was removed during initial debridement, as it was nonviable, and antibiotic cement beads were used for dead space management with later conversion to a block spacer. She was placed in a knee-spanning external fixator for staged treatment of her injury. The plan was to return to the operating room for soft tissue coverage and definitive fixation of her fractures. CT scanning was also done to better characterize the joint involvement and the "personality" of the fracture (Fig. 6.2a–d).

She underwent four subsequent debridements, and was 10 days from initial injury at the time of definitive open reduction and internal fixation (ORIF) with circular external fixation and gastrocnemius flap coverage (Fig. 6.3a–c). An anterolateral approach and arthrotomy were used to elevate the joint depression, bone-graft the defect, and place rafting screws across the tibial plateau (Fig. 6.4a–f). This was then closed, and the plastic surgery team provided soft tissue coverage with a gastrocnemius rotational flap and skin grafting. After this was complete, in the same operative setting, we completed our fixation by applying a circular external fixation device (Taylor Spatial Frame, Smith and Nephew, Memphis, TN). This was done with a hybrid technique, utilizing both tensioned wires and half pins (and incorporating the pins in the distal shaft from the spanning fixator). We replaced the antibiotic beads with an antibiotic cement spacer block, with plans for later removal and autogenous bone grafting of the metaphyseal bone defect. Due to her soft tissue injury, the ringed external fixator was chosen as an optimal construct to allow for early knee mobilization and also to allow for wound access and flap monitoring.

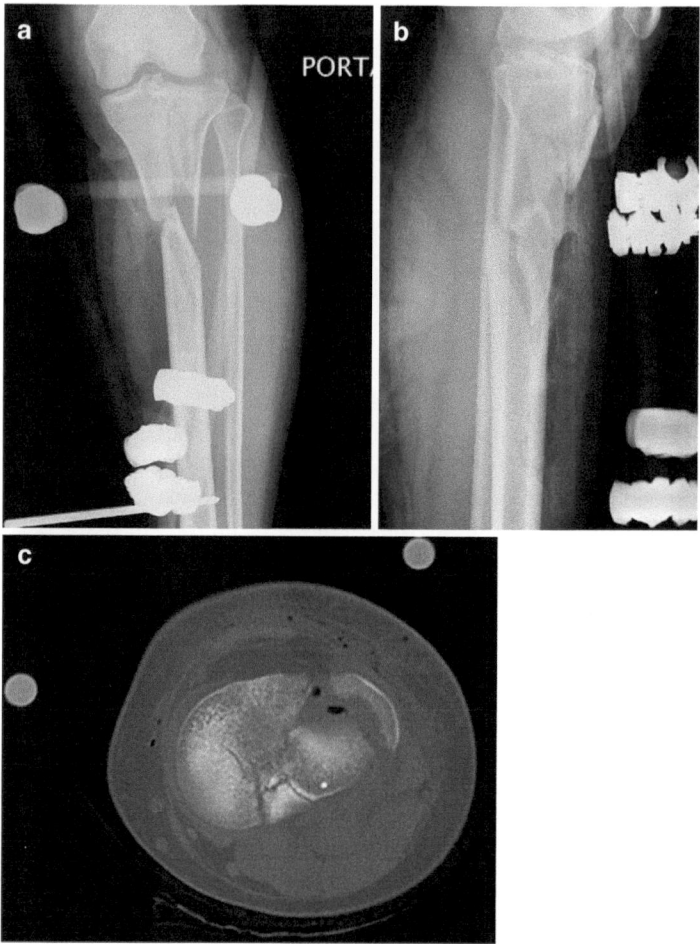

Fig. 6.2 After debridement, spanning external fixation, and antibiotic bead placement (**a**, **b**) Postoperative radiographs after temporary external fixator placement. Fracture length is restored. (**c**, **d**) Axial and coronal CT images demonstrated that the fracture is bicondylar and with significant metaphyseal-diaphyseal dissociation. (**e**) Intraoperative photograph after preliminary debridement demonstrating partial wound closure with a concomitant large area of soft tissue loss. Antibiotic cement beads are placed in the bone defect

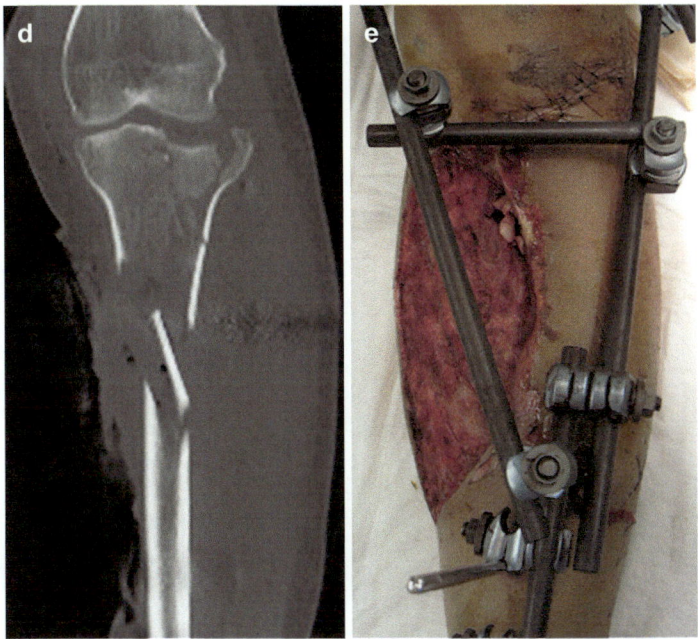

Fig. 6.2 (continued)

Intraoperative Tips and Tricks for Reduction

This particular case involves a relatively simple joint depression and mild-moderately displaced condyles of the proximal tibia. When treating this or a more complex articular fracture with ring fixators, adhering to basic AO principles still applies:

1. *Anatomic reduction*: Regardless of the implant choice (i.e., plates vs ring fixator), definitive management should still strive to achieve an anatomic or near-anatomic reduction of the articular surface. It is important to also restore the mechanical axis through the knee, and thereby the lower extremity.

   Anatomic reduction of the articular surface in any tibial plateau fracture usually involves open reduction, elevation of the depressed portion, reduction and compression of the split

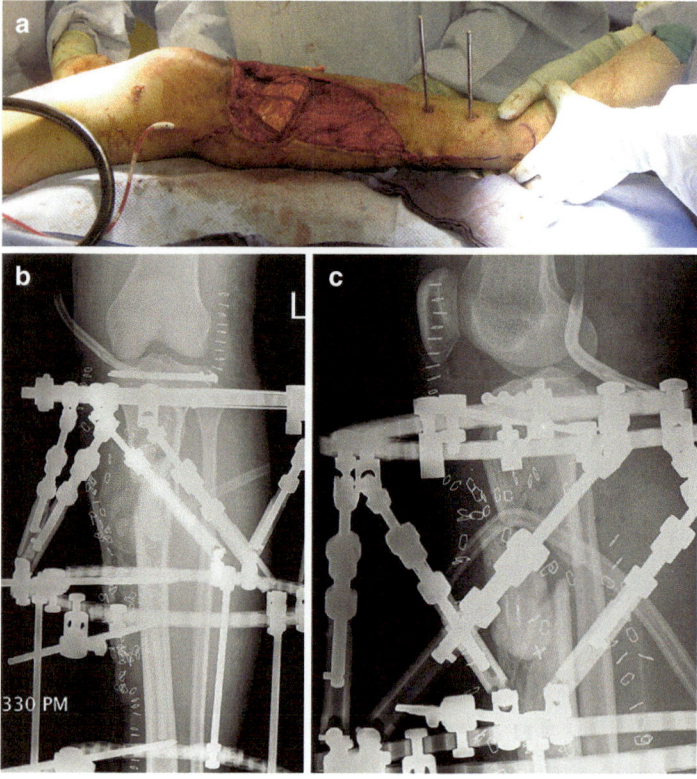

Fig. 6.3 Flap coverage, ORIF with circular fixation, and antibiotic cement block spacer placement done. (**a**) Intraoperative photograph demonstrating the soft tissue coverage with a medial gastrocnemius flap. (**b**, **c**) AP and lateral postoperative radiographs demonstrating satisfactory articular and axial alignment with the cement spacer visible, articular rafting screws, and the circular external fixation hybrid device with both tensioned wires and half pins

condylar fragments, and both subchondral and interfragmentary screw support.

In most bicondylar fracture patterns, reduction and fixation of the medial condyle is done first. This is then followed by addressing the depression, and finally the lateral split. In this particular case, the medial fragment was an extremely large fragment with minimal displacement. We therefore were able to control this fragment with a periarticular reduction forceps without difficulty. Our first step for definitive reduction was to perform an anterolateral arthrotomy to gain direct visualization of the joint depression. Bone tamps were utilized to elevate the articular surface, and provisional Kirschner pins were used to maintain the reduction. Bone-graft substitute was utilized to support the depression; then, the split was reduced and compressed with the periarticular reduction forceps, and 3.5 mm screws were placed in the subchondral position to support the depression (Fig. 6.4a–d).

2. *Stable fixation*: General principles for achieving stable fixation with ring fixators were applied. We placed the tensioned wires

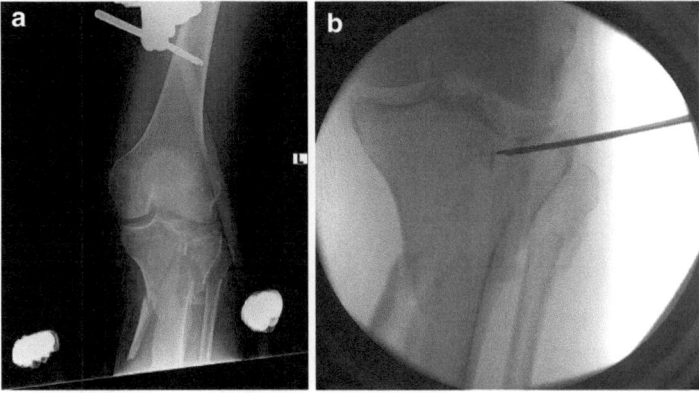

Fig. 6.4 A separate case is presented for comparison and illustration of technical points. A 62-year-old gentleman with peripheral vascular disease, with a high-energy closed Schatzker VI tibial plateau fracture with severe blistering and soft tissue injury, was treated with spanning external fixation. This was treated definitively with ORIF of the lateral depression and condyles, and circular external fixation. (**a**) AP radiograph after spanning external fixation demonstrating more of a prototypical Schatzker VI injury than the main case discussed in this chapter. (**b–d**) An anterolateral approach and arthrotomy was performed. Intraoperative images show elevation of the joint depression, then provisional wire fixation of the major portion of the joint depression. (**e**) The circular fixator is shown with a partial ring at the level of the knee and two rings spanning the distal bone segment. Note that the two distal half-pins were initially from the spanning ex fix, and were incorporated into the circular fixator. (**f**) Postop radiograph demonstrating ORIF with bone grafting, rafting screws, and circular fixation with tensioned wires in the proximal segment

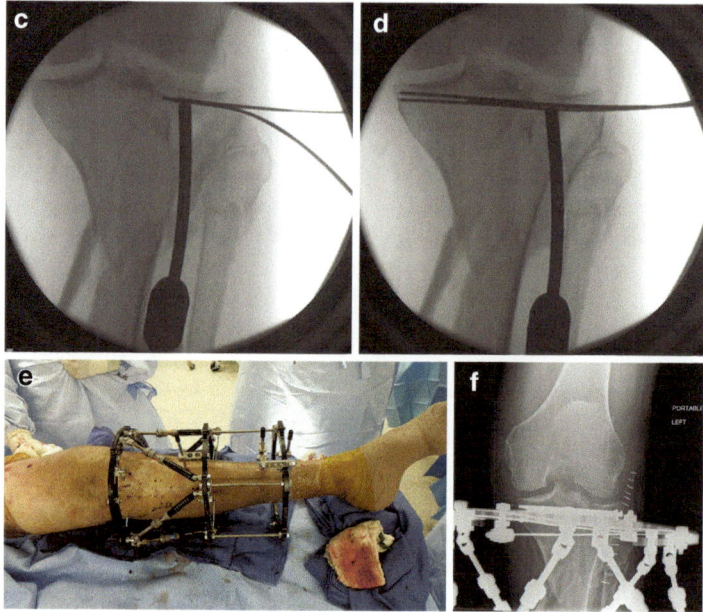

Fig. 6.4 (continued)

at a wide angle with respect to each other proximally (case example using a different patient – Fig. 6.4e). It is also critical to place the pins distal to the capsular reflection to prevent late joint sepsis from an infected pin site. The fixators (and rings) are all placed perpendicular to the tibial shaft. Two rings were used in the distal segment to maximize stability. In this case, we also utilized Taylor Spatial struts (Smith and Nephew, Memphis, TN) in order to help facilitate the metaphyseal fracture reduction. Ring size was chosen as a compromise between stability (more stable with a smaller ring) and soft tissue access (improved with a larger ring).

3. *Preservation of the blood supply*: This is arguably easier to achieve with the use of ring fixators, compared with plates and screws. We try to avoid unnecessary stripping of bone fragments, particularly in this case with severe soft tissue injury from the initial trauma.

4. *Early mobilization*: The ring fixator allows early motion of the knee joint, although extreme flexion is difficult due to pin impingement posteriorly. In this particular case, and in most bicondylar tibial plateau fractures treated with this device, early motion should be possible. With poor bone quality, severe comminution, significant concomitant ligamentous injury, or patient compliance problems, stabilization across the knee joint can be achieved by utilizing a hinged ring fixator. This allows dynamic distraction (if needed) as well as improved varus and valgus stability to external forces. We frequently utilize the pins from the initial spanning (static) external fixator to incorporate into the hinged frame. The hinged component proximal to the tibia can then be removed frequently after 4–6 weeks.

Postoperative Rehab Protocol

The articular component of this tibial plateau fracture dictated non-weight-bearing period of 3 months to allow for bony healing at the joint. Range of motion began immediately postoperatively with CPM and with passive range of motion exercises, with supervised physical therapy. The ringed fixator construct allowed for knee motion and wound care while maintaining stability of the metadiaphyseal dissociation.

Follow-Up

The patient was lost to follow-up for several weeks, and her visiting nurses were unable to access her home initially. She then returned to the emergency room with wound drainage, and maggots were found over a small portion of her gastrocnemius flap.

She required two debridements as an inpatient, followed by local wound care as an outpatient (Fig. 6.5). The planned bone grafting for her segmental bone loss was further complicated by early pregnancy, which was diagnosed during this admission. After consultation with OB/Gyn, the decision was made, at 6 months postinjury (during her second trimester), to proceed with

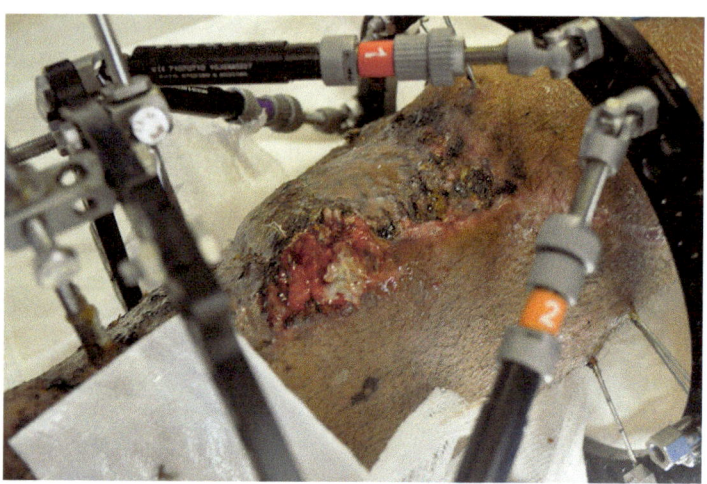

Fig. 6.5 Partial flap necrosis with maggots discovered in wound. This was treated with operative debridement, local wound care, and no change in any of the fixation

bone grafting. The cement block was removed, and autologous (femoral reaming) bone grafting was done utilizing the RIA system (DepuySynthes, Paoli, PA). Iliac crest was not utilized, to avoid any potential injury to the fetus. The bone grafting would ordinarily have been done 4–6 weeks after cement block placement. Her ringed external fixator was maintained through the course of her pregnancy and removed after delivery. It was felt that she was safer to be fully weight-bearing with the device in place rather than removing it and either imposing weight-bearing restrictions or risking refracture (Fig. 6.6).

She had successful union of her fracture, 3 months after bone grafting, and had a 2.5 year period free of infection or wound complication. She returned to clinic, after a period of more than 1.5 years (4 years from initial injury), with drainage and redness near a previous pin site at the anterolateral tibia, close to her rafting screws. A superficial abscess was noted, and operative debridement was performed including screw removal. However,

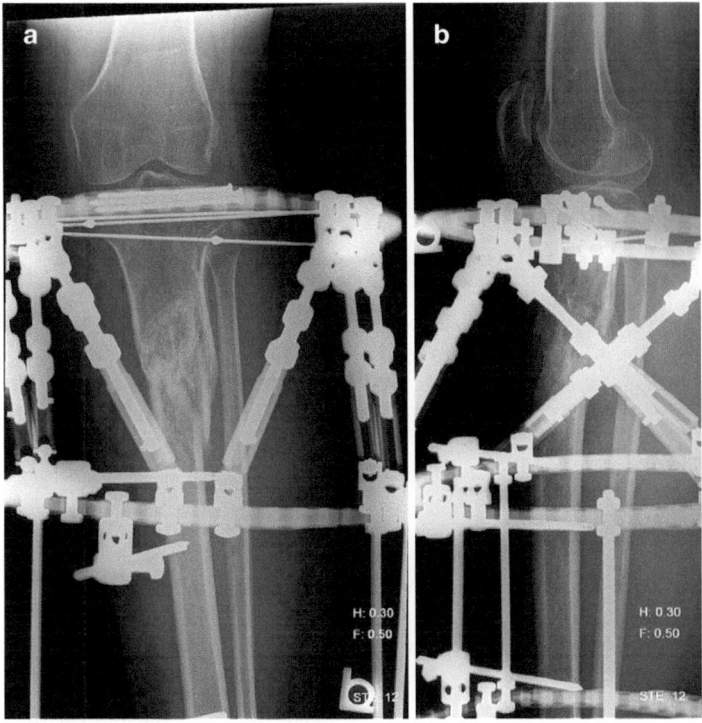

Fig. 6.6 Fracture healing. (**a**, **b**) Bony union noted on AP and lateral radiographs at 5 months after bone grafting and 11 months after initial injury

no obvious deep abscess, loose screws, or bone necrosis were noted. She has had no further complications to this point (Fig. 6.7).

Salient Points/Pearls

- Using a ring fixator is an exacting procedure and requires commitment from both the surgeon and the patient.
- It allows for treatment of complex tibial fractures, both open and closed, and also for nonunion and bone transport if needed.
- Immediate weight-bearing is permissible with secure fixation.

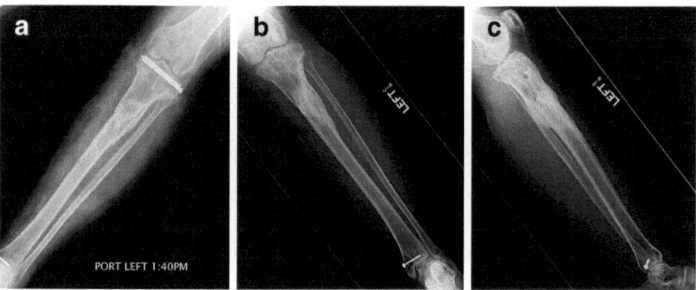

Fig. 6.7 Presentation with localized infection anterolaterally at 39 months postoperatively. (**a**) AP radiograph demonstrating a healed tibia with retained rafting screws proximally. (**b, c**) Radiographs after incision and drainage, removal of implants, and exploration of the tibia and medullary canal. No obvious infection of the screws or bone was noted. The lateral image here shows a potential area of bone lysis, which was explored, but no fluid collection or bone necrosis was found. She has remained complication-free since then

- This can also be used in the presence of infection and may help treat the same.
- Soft tissue management including flap placement may be challenging, as the bars may need to be repositioned for the same.
- Time in external fixation can be shortened by nailing the tibia, once lengthening is completed or infection is controlled.

Further Reading

Ariffin HM, et al. Modified hybrid fixator for high-energy Schatzker V and VI tibial plateau fractures. Strategies Trauma Limb Reconstr. 2011;6(1):21–6.

Mankar SH, et al. Outcome of complex tibial plateau fractures treated with external fixator. Indian J Orthop. 2012;46(5):570–4.

Babis GC, et al. High energy tibial plateau fractures treated with hybrid external fixation. J Orthop Surg Res. 2011;6:35.

Kummer FJ, et al. Biomechanics of the Ilizarov external fixator. Clin Orthop Relat Res. 1992;280:11–4.

Horesh Z, et al. Treatment of complex tibial plateau fracture with Ilizarov external fixation and minimal open surgical procedure. JBJS Br. 2008;90-B pp 514.

Benirschke SK, Agnew SG, Mayo KA, Santoro VM, Henley MB. Immediate internal fixation of open, complex tibial plateau fractures: treatment by a standard protocol. J Orthop Trauma. 1992;6:78–86.

Chapter 7
Bicondylar Tibial Plateau Fracture with Compartment Syndrome

Jennifer M. Bauer and Hassan R. Mir

Case Presentation

A 34-year-old man sustained a closed right tibial plateau fracture as the passenger in a golf cart rollover accident. He was transferred from an outside hospital and evaluated in the emergency room 6 h after injury. At the time, his leg compartments were but compressible, with normal distal sensation and pulses, and no pain with passive stretch.

Injury Films

Injury films including anteroposterior (AP) and lateral views show a right Schatzker VI tibial plateau fracture (Fig. 7.1). Computed tomography (CT) is usually obtained on these injuries for more detailed information on articular involvement and comminution,

J.M. Bauer, MD, MS (✉)
Vanderbilt University, Nashville, TN, USA
e-mail: hmirwvu@aol.com

H.R. Mir, MD, MBA, FACS
University of South Florida, Tampa, FL, USA

© Springer International Publishing Switzerland 2016   85
N.C. Tejwani (ed.), *Fractures of the Tibia: A Clinical Casebook*,
DOI 10.1007/978-3-319-21774-1_7

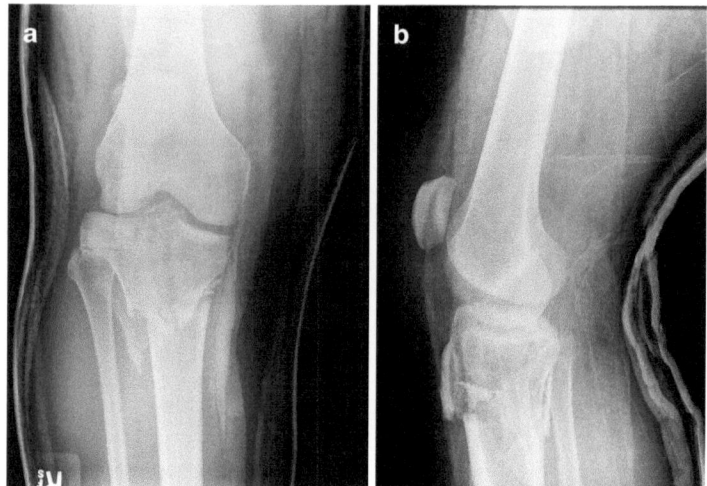

Fig. 7.1 (**a**) (AP) (**b**) (lat): initial films

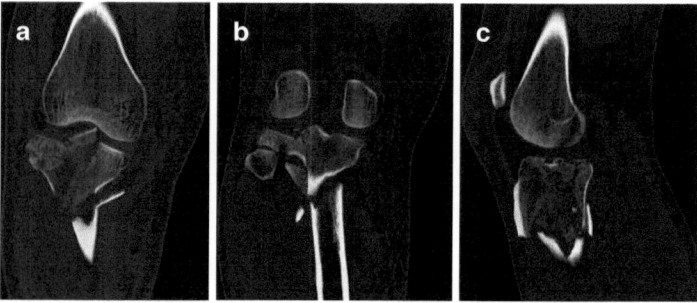

Fig. 7.2 CT right tibia, coronal (**a**) anterior cut; (**b**) posterior cut; (**c**) sagittal cut

and is usually obtained after initial spanning external fixation for restoration of length and alignment, which allows for better imaging. This patient had preoperative CT scans, which show intraarticular involvement and metaphyseal comminution, including a separate tibial tubercle fragment (Fig. 7.2).

Treatment and Timing of Surgery

The patient underwent serial exams on the night of admission, which showed worsening signs of compartment syndrome, including increasing pain and medication requirements; swollen, firm compartments; pain on passive stretch of toes and ankle. He was taken urgently to the operating room for leg fasciotomies and placement of spanning external fixation.

Surgical Tact

Positioning

Supine, with a bump under ipsilateral hip. The leg is elevated on a radiolucent ramp to allow for lateral fluoroscopic imaging, with clearance of the contralateral limb.

Approach

Four-compartment leg fasciotomies can be performed with either a single lateral incision or dual medial and lateral incisions. Preoperative planning based on the CT determined the need for bicondylar plating, and thus a two-incision fasciotomy was performed with placement of the incisions to allow for staged definitive fixation through the same approaches.

Fixation

A knee-spanning external fixator was applied with 5 mm Schanz pins in a multiplanar fashion, ensuring restoration of length, alignment, and rotation (Fig. 7.3). Again, final fixation must be considered with tibial pins kept out of the zone of injury and also future definitive fixation.

Fasciotomy wounds were dressed with negative-pressure dressings (VAC), with the use of narrow sponge strips and staples to

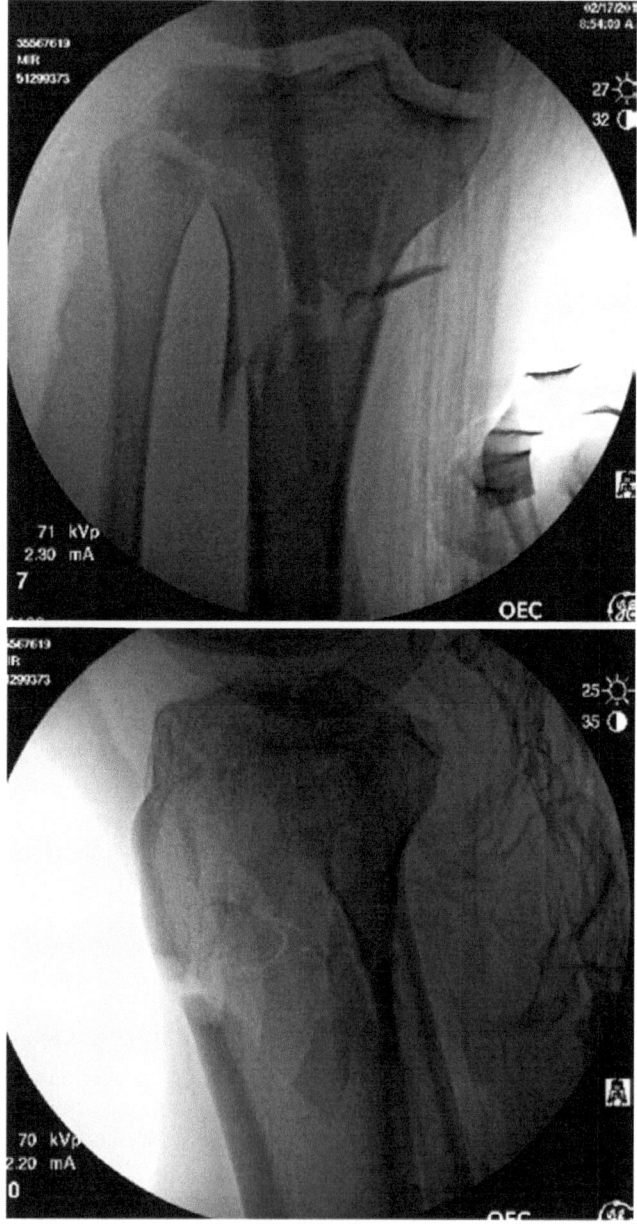

Fig. 7.3 Intraoperative fluoroscopy, reduced in external fixator

avoid excessive gapping of the skin edges. A long leg posterior splint was applied to further stabilize the limb.

Postoperative Plan

The patient was kept non-weight-bearing on his right leg, with strict instructions for elevation of the injured extremity above chest level. Soft tissue swelling was checked daily until the wounds were likely to close primarily. This can typically be done 3–7 days after the initial procedure, and if unable to be closed primarily after a sufficient delay to allow for resolution of edema, skin grafting is warranted.

Definitive Fixation and Timing of Surgery

On postoperative day 5, the patient was taken back to the OR for definitive fixation and closure of his fasciotomy wounds.

Surgical Tact

Positioning

Supine, with a bump under the ipsilateral hip to allow for neutral positioning of leg. The leg is elevated on a radiolucent ramp to allow for lateral fluoroscopic imaging, with clearance of the contralateral limb. A small radiolucent towel bump is used to provide knee flexion as necessary throughout the procedure.

Approach

The medial and lateral fasciotomy wounds were extended proximally to gain access to the tibial plateau. All muscles appeared viable in all the four leg compartments. On the lateral side, a submeniscal arthrotomy was used to visualize the joint surface. On the medial side, protection of the superficial medial collateral ligament is paramount, while the pes anserine tendons may be tenotomized with subsequent repair if necessary.

Fracture Reduction and Fixation

A femoral distractor was utilized with a distal femoral Schanz pin, placed through extension of the lateral incision, and a new tibial Schanz pin. The posteromedial fracture fragments were provisionally reduced and pinned, followed by nonlocking buttress fixation. A submeniscal arthrotomy allowed direct visualization of the lateral joint surface to address the joint depression. The lateral condyle was reduced and then secured to the metadiaphysis with a periarticular contoured variable angle lateral locking plate, with all nonlocking screws utilized.

An additional one-third tubular plate was used to secure the tibial tubercle fragment. Intraoperative fluoroscopy as well as direct joint visualization and knee ROM proved appropriate implant placement and construct stability.

The tourniquet was inflated for 120 min, let down for 20 min, and then reinflated for 30 min to minimize edema and assist in primary closure of the fasciotomy wounds under minimal tension.

Postoperative Plan

Immediate postoperative films were performed (Fig. 7.4). Range of motion exercises started at 1 week postoperatively, and all sutures were removed by 3 weeks postoperatively. After 12 weeks, the patient was progressed through a physical therapy program to full weight-bearing. Clinical and radiographic follow-up were continued for 1 full year.

Outcomes

Follow-up radiographs showed progression to union with no loss of fixation throughout follow-up (Fig. 7.5). The patient returned to work at 6 months after injury. At 1-year follow-up, the patient has no pain and no plans for hardware removal.

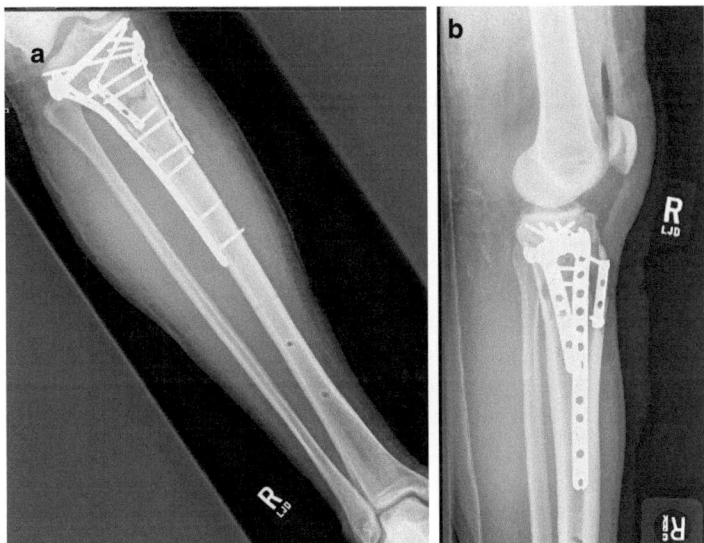

Fig. 7.4 Postoperative X-rays after ORIF (**a**) AP and (**b**) lateral

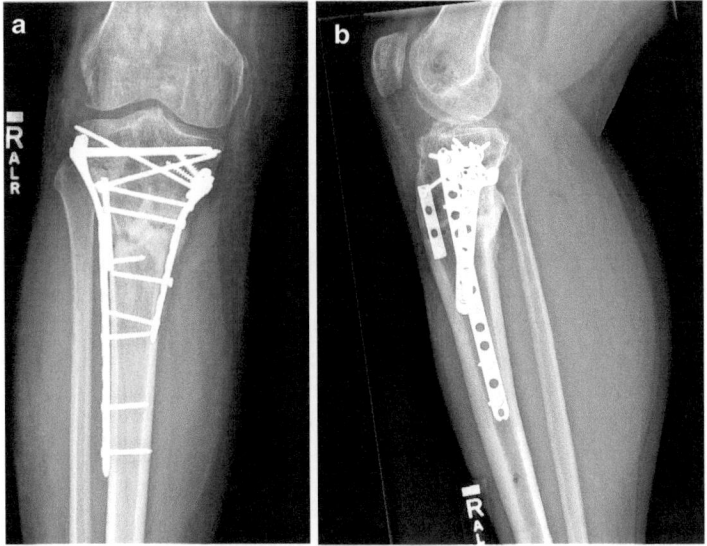

Fig. 7.5 Final follow-up films (**a**) AP and (**b**) lateral

Complications

A postoperative tourniquet neuropraxia completely resolved by 3 months postoperatively. Two small areas of wound dehiscence after suture removal were successfully treated with local wound care.

Salient Points/Pearls

- Serial compartment examinations should be performed on all high-energy bicondylar tibial fractures; there is a 14.5 % incidence of compartment syndrome [1]. Compartment pressure measurements are controversial and are not necessary in patients with unaltered mental status and positive clinical findings.
- The average interval between external fixation and definitive treatment is 9 days [1], thus achieving anatomic length with the initial operation as imperative. Schanz pins should be kept out of the zone of definitive fixation when possible.
- Infection rate for bicondylar tibial plateau fractures has been reported up to 14.2 %, with compartment syndrome as a risk factor for infection [2].
- An equivalent infection risk has been demonstrated between single-incision and dual-incision fasciotomies for tibial fractures treated with either a nail or plate [3].
- The surgeon must confirm complete release of all the four leg compartments, with either technique utilized (single or dual incision). Care must be taken to plan the incision(s), based on the approach(es) planned for definitive fixation. If dual plating is needed, a two-incision fasciotomy can be performed with placement of the incisions to allow for staged definitive fixation through the same approaches. Alternatively, a single-incision fasciotomy technique can be used with the incision placed more posterolaterally to allow for the surgical fixation to occur through separate anterolateral and medial incisions.
- Timing of definitive fixation and fasciotomy closure is case dependent. In some cases, the fasciotomy wounds can be closed/skin grafted, and then the definitive fixation can be

delayed until edema has subsided, and the surgical fixation approaches can be safely performed. For others, fixation can be performed at the time of skin closure/coverage.

- Dual plating is commonly necessary, with screws acting to support articular reconstruction and plating with a balanced construct for limb alignment. Careful preoperative planning ensures that fixation constructs will address all unstable articular and metadiaphyseal fracture fragments.
- Locking screws are necessary for severe comminution or poor bone quality.
- Preoperative understanding of the articular involvement and intraoperative direct visualization allows for anatomic articular reduction, which has a significant association with better long-term function [4].

References

1. Barei DP, et al. Complications associated with internal fixation of high-energy bicondylar tibial plateau fractures utilizing a two-incision technique. J Orthop Trauma. 2004;18(10):649–57.
2. Morris BJ, et al. Risk factors of infection after ORIF of bicondylar tibial plateau fractures. J Orthop Trauma. 2013;27(9):e196–200.
3. Bible JE, McClure DJ, Mir HR. Analysis of single-incision versus dual-incision fasciotomy for tibial fractures with acute compartment syndrome. J Orthop Trauma. 2013;27(11):607–11.
4. Barei DP, et al. Functional outcomes of severe bicondylar tibial plateau fractures treated with dual incisions and medial and lateral plates. J Bone Joint Surg Am. 2006;88(8):1713–21.

Part II
Treatment of Tibia Shaft Fractures

Chapter 8
Proximal Third Tibia Fracture Treated with Intramedullary Nailing

Kostas Triantafillou and Edward Perez

Clinical Scenario

CH is a 50-year-old male pedestrian struck by a car with a chief complaint of right leg pain. Given the mechanism of injury, he was brought in by ambulance as trauma activation and evaluated using the Advanced Trauma Life Support (ATLS) protocol. Subsequent secondary and tertiary surveys were notable for an isolated closed fracture of the right proximal tibia without neurovascular deficit (Fig. 8.1a, b). He was placed in a long-leg splint for stabilization until definitive fixation; his compartments were serially monitored by clinical exam; and a CT scan evaluation for fracture extension into the tibial plateau was negative (Fig. 8.2a, b).

Treatment Algorithm

With few exceptions, displaced extraarticular proximal tibial shaft fractures are treated operatively due to the poorly tolerated effects of malunion. Evaluation of the status of the soft tissues is the most

K. Triantafillou (✉) • E. Perez
Department of Orthopaedic Trauma,
Campbell Clinic Orthopaedics, Memphis, TN, USA
e-mail: Kostas.m.triantafillou@gmail.com

© Springer International Publishing Switzerland 2016
N.C. Tejwani (ed.), *Fractures of the Tibia: A Clinical Casebook*,
DOI 10.1007/978-3-319-21774-1_8

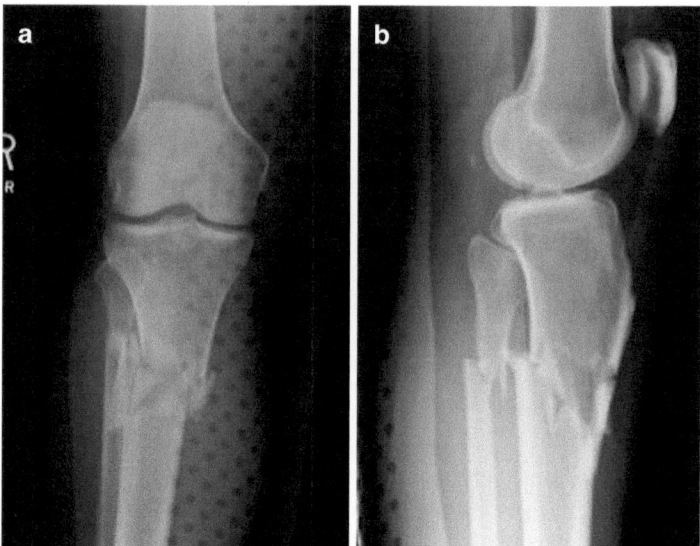

Fig. 8.1 Injury films (**a**, **b**): Injury films demonstrate a proximal third tibial fracture with a long proximal segment amenable to tibial intramedullary nailing. It is important to be familiar with the interlocking hole distances of the nail available at your institution, and preoperative templating is encouraged

important factor when selecting treatment options [1]. Fractures with minimal soft-tissue injury, which include closed fractures with minimal swelling, are amenable to plate fixation, multiplanar fine-wire external fixation, or intramedullary fixation. The choice of fixation is determined by the surgeon's familiarity with the technique and the length of the proximal fragment. Longer proximal fragments that can accommodate three interlocking screws are preferably fixed using intramedullary implants, whereas a very short proximal fragment may require fine wire fixation or plating. Fractures with severe soft-tissue injury, including open fractures, compartment syndrome, or vascular injury repair, should be initially treated with temporizing external fixation until soft-tissue coverage or adequate healing has occurred.

CH has a closed fracture with minimal soft-tissue injury, and the proximal fragment is long enough to accommodate three interlocking screws. Thus, intramedullary fixation is the preferred treatment option.

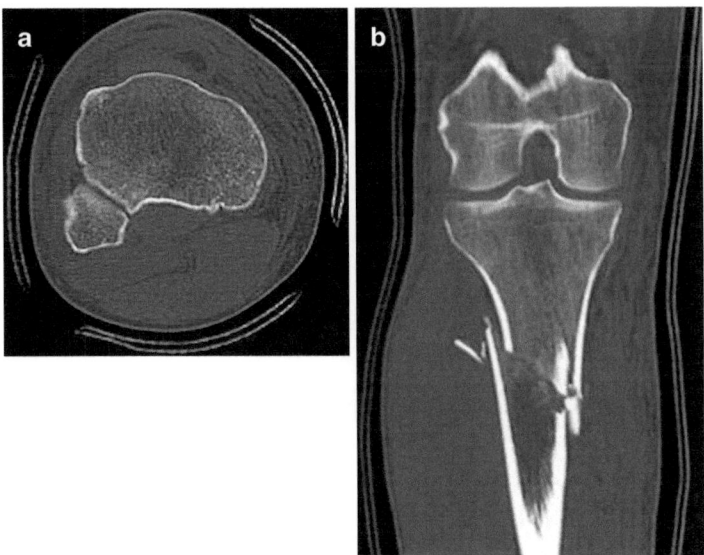

Fig. 8.2 CT scans (**a**, **b**): Preoperative computed tomography is encouraged in proximal third tibial fractures to prevent displacement of an unrecognized tibial plateau fracture during nail insertion

Treatment Considerations with Proximal Third Tibial Nailing

Intramedullary nailing of proximal third tibial fractures was initially discouraged in favor of plate osteosynthesis or external fixation, due to the observation that proximal tibial nailing commonly resulted in apex anterior and valgus malalignment [2]. Diaphyseal fractures of the tibia are reduced by the isthmal fit of the nail; however, proximal tibial fractures are not corrected this way due to the discrepancy of a relatively small nail within a voluminous soft cancellous metaphysis. Therefore, the reduction of a proximal tibial fracture relies on a perfect start point in line with the anatomic axis of the tibia. A start point that is too medial, resulting in a lateral nail trajectory, often occurs due to the constraints of patellar tendon or a deficient lateral cortex (Fig. 8.3b). A start point that is too anterior, resulting in a posterior nail trajectory, often occurs due to the constraint of the patella or the deforming forces of the

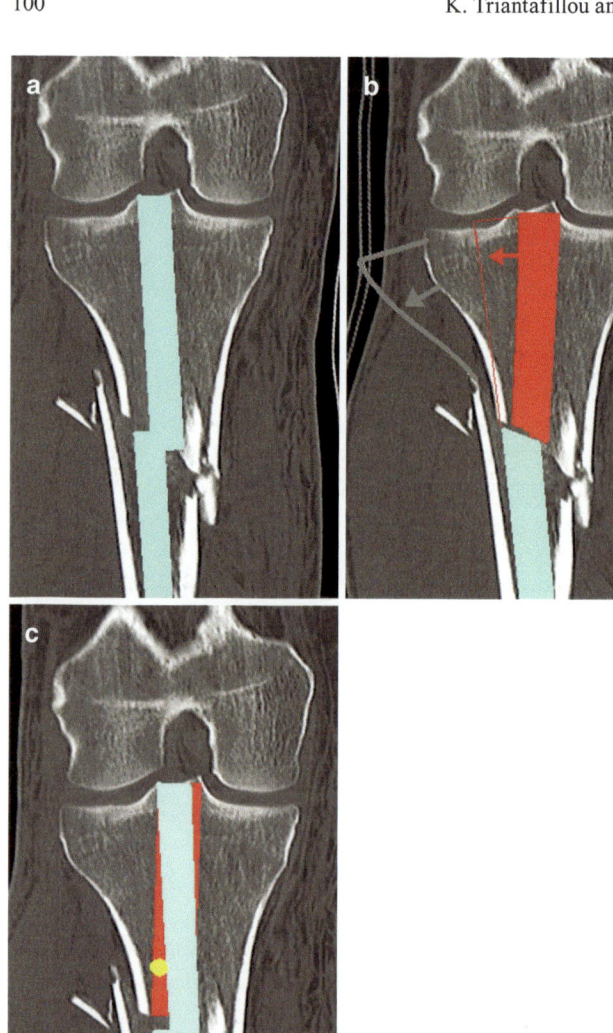

extensor mechanism with the knee flexed. As a result, when the nail abuts the posterior and lateral cortices of the distal fragment, the nail "straightens" along the anatomic axis of the tibia, resulting in a vector that levers the proximal fragment into procurvatum (apex anterior) and valgus deformity.

Intraoperative Tips and Tricks for Reduction/ Fixation

Given the advantages of fixation with tibial nailing, several techniques were developed to overcome the difficulties associated with proximal tibial nailing. The use of minifragmentary provisional fixation was described as an adjunct, which facilitated proximal fragment alignment at the expense of an additional incision and disruption of the healing milieu. However, the force vector of a nail with an aberrant trajectory often overcame the reduction achieved with provisional fixation. A lateral parapatellar approach was described to help facilitate an anatomic start point in the coronal plane, but does not address sagittal malalignment. Therefore, techniques which facilitated optimal start point and trajectory became the workhorse for anatomic reduction of proximal tibial fractures with intramedullary fixation.

Fig. 8.3 Technical figures (**a**): Appropriate trajectory within the proximal segment will prevent varus and valgus malposition during nail insertion. It is important to note that prior to reaming, the fracture must be reduced to prevent eccentric reaming of the cortices at the fracture site, risking malreduction. (**b**) A lateral trajectory will result in a valgus vector during nail insertion. (**c**) A Poller screw, as demonstrated by the *yellow circle*, may be placed distally within a reamed canal with an aberrant lateral trajectory with a correct starting point. This requires removal of the reduction tool or nail. Of note, a Poller screw will correct coronal plane malalignment, but may result in mild translation if the combination of a medial starting point and a lateral trajectory is present

A semiextended medial parapatellar arthrotomy, an adoption of the approach used for total knee arthroplasty, facilitates the appropriate lateral and high start point, because it allows for lateral subluxation of the patella. This removes the constraint of the patella and tendon against the starting wire, allowing the surgeon to place the start point more posteriorly and laterally and direct the starting wire more anteriorly and medially, respectively [3]. This technique has been modified so as to be performed via an extraarticular approach [4], thus reducing the risk of cartilage damage and preventing retained intraarticular reamings. Lateral retraction of the patella is performed following parapatellar retinacular incision to the level of the quad tendon with care not to violate the synovium. The infrapatellar fat pad is then sharply detached at its inferior margin, exposing the anatomic start point.

The semiextended suprapatellar approach, which requires the use of special instrumentation, was developed to capitalize on the advantages of the open semiextended techniques without the theoretic morbidity of a larger incision. Though long-term functional outcomes are not established, short-term results indicate minimal risk of damage of the patellofemoral joint with the use of the suprapatellar guide [5].

Pöller, or blocking screws, can be used as an adjunct to guide nail trajectory by reducing the volume within the metaphysis through which the nail can pass, and also prevent late malalignment by preventing nail migration [6]. The screws are positioned posteriorly and laterally within the proximal segment adjacent to the nail path. More simply, blocking screws are placed on the concavity of the deformity. Interlocking screws or 3.2 mm pins may be used to prevent bending or breakage associated with the use of drill bits or smaller diameter screws.

A combination of techniques is sometimes required for very proximal tibial fractures or those with proximal extension. The surgeon should use any of the techniques to ensure proper nail start point and trajectory if he/she is to prevent the typical pitfalls associated with intramedullary nailing of proximal tibial fractures.

Given the advantages of semiextended approaches for proximal tibial shaft fractures, the operative surgeon chose to utilize a medial parapatellar arthrotomy in the case of CH. After the start point was selected, and the opening reamer was used with care to protect articular surface, a reduction tool was used through the proximal segment to pass the guide wire. Subsequently, it was noted that the opening reamer trajectory was oriented more laterally than desired, with the concern that nail insertion would force the proximal segment into valgus. Therefore, a Pöller, or blocking screw, was inserted laterally to prevent valgus malalignment (see Fig. 8.4a, b). It is important to note that a blocking screw used to correct an incorrect nail trajectory must be within the aberrant path, and therefore the nail or reduction tool must be drawn back before placement of the Pöller screw (Fig. 8.3c). This is in contrast to a blocking screw used to prevent late migration, which can be done adjacent to a well-placed nail.

Postoperative Protocols

Proximal third tibial fractures are axially unstable due to the lack of interference fit. Although Poller screws and interlocking screws

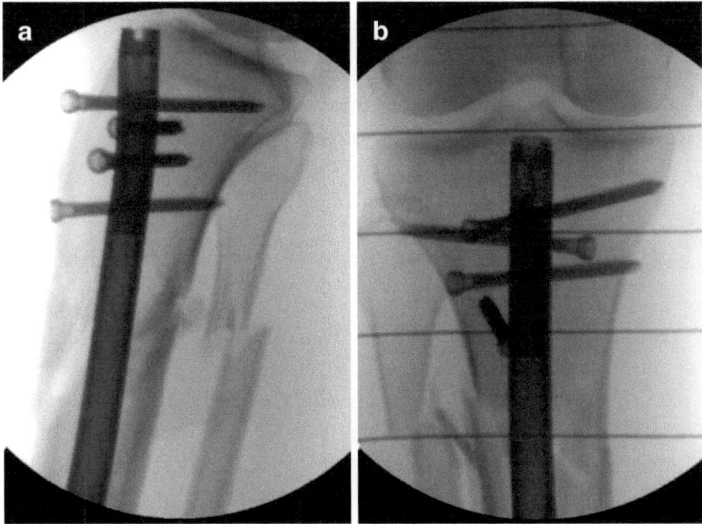

Fig. 8.4 Intraoperative photos/flouros (**a, b**): Intraoperative fluoroscopy demonstrating lateral and distal placement of a Poller screw in the sagittal plane

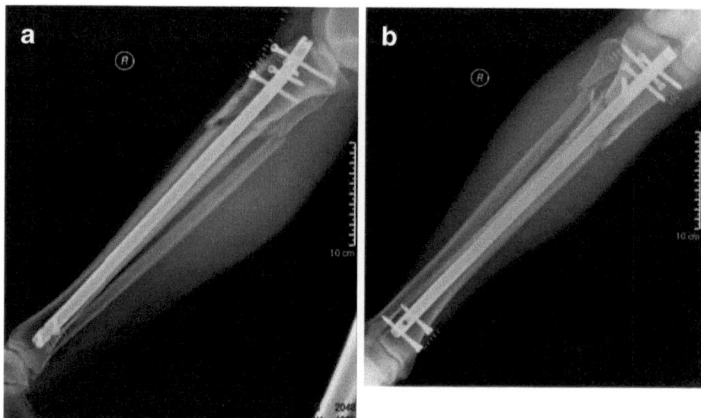

Fig. 8.5 Postop films (**a**, **b**): Immediate postoperative films demonstrating anatomic coronal alignment achieved by correction of a lateral trajectory with a lateral Poller screw, and anatomic sagittal alignment facilitated by a semiextended approach

oriented orthogonally may help prevent late migration, it is unclear if they provide enough multiplanar stability in the cancellous metaphysis for early weight bearing. Therefore, weight-bearing is restricted for 4–6 weeks until early callous appears, and then advanced as tolerated. Range of motion exercises are begun and encouraged immediately postoperatively (Fig. 8.5).

Follow-Up with Union/Complications

Postoperatively, CH went on to clinical and radiographic union at 5 months. Of note, CH had late migration in the sagittal plane resulting in mild procurvatum deformity, which was within acceptable alignment and was not expected to affect the clinical outcome (Fig. 8.6a, b). Prevention of late migration could have been accomplished via positional screws adjacent to the nail following nail placement laterally, and in CH's case, posteriorly.

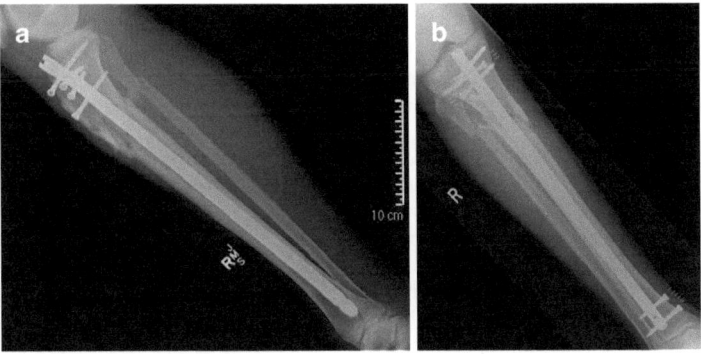

Fig. 8.6 Follow-up films (**a, b**): Note maintenance of varus and valgus alignment with mild late procurvatum deformity at 3 months. Placement of a posterior positional Pöller screw may have prevented this late deformity

Anecdotally, and in the case of CH, anterior knee pain is reduced using semiextended techniques for reasons that are unclear. The nailing of proximal tibial third fractures, though more technically challenging, can result in superior outcomes if done appropriately using any combination of techniques used to ensure proper alignment and prevention of late nail migration.

Pearls/Salient Points

- Proximal third tibial fractures are difficult to nail and have a high percentage of malunion (varus and extension of the proximal fragment) if not reduced
- Reduction before nailing and maintenance until locking screws are inserted is important to achieve optimal outcomes
- Multiple techniques including lateral starting point, semiextended, suprapatellar nailing, use of blocking screws or plates and/or ex ternal fixators for provisional fixation may be utilized
- Proximal articular extension, if present, should be fixed using either supplemental screws or plate along with nailing.

References

1. Bono CM, Levine RG, Rao JP, Behrens FF. Nonarticular proximal tibia fractures: treatment options and decision making. J Am Acad Orthop Surg. 2001;9:176.
2. Lang GL, Cohen BE, Bosse MJ, Kellam JF. Proximal third tibial shaft fractures. Should they be nailed? Clin Orthop Relat Res. 1995;315:64–74.
3. Tornetta P, Collins E. Semiextended position of intramedullary nailing of the proximal tibia. Clin Orthop Relat Res. 1996;328:185–9.
4. Kubiak EN, Widmer BJ, Horwitz DS. Extra-articular technique for semiextended tibial nailing. J Orthop Trauma. 2010;24(11):704–8.
5. Sanders RW, DiPasquale TG, Jordan CJ, Arrington JA, Sagi HC. Semiextended intramedullary nailing of the tibia using a suprapatellar approach: radiographic results and clinical outcomes at a minimum of 12 months follow-up. J Orthop Trauma. 2014;28(5):245–55.
6. Krettek C, Miclau T, Schandelmaier P, Stephan C, Möhlmann U, Tscherne H. The mechanical effect of blocking screws ("Poller screws") in stabilizing tibia fractures with short proximal or distal fragments after insertion of small-diameter intramedullary nails. J Orthop Trauma. 1999;13:550–3.

Chapter 9
Proximal Tibia Fracture Treated with Plate and Screws

Milan K. Sen

Case Presentation

A 45-year-old male accidentally drove his truck into the back of an 18 wheel semi-trailer truck. He sustained bilateral lower extremity injuries including closed fractures of the right proximal tibia and ipsilateral patella.

Injury Films

Injury films (Figs. 9.1 and 9.2) demonstrate a displaced oblique proximal tibia fracture and a comminuted patella fracture. There appears to be undisplaced fracture lines extending into the knee joint. CT scan confirms the X-ray findings (Figs. 9.3 and 9.4).

M.K. Sen, MD, FRCSC, FAAOS
Division of Orthopedic Surgery, Orthopedic Trauma Jacobi Medical Center, Albert Einstein College of Medicine Orthopedic Trauma, Wrist, and Elbow Surgeon, Gotham City Orthopedics LLC
New York, NY, USA
e-mail: msenmd@gmail.com

© Springer International Publishing Switzerland 2016   107
N.C. Tejwani (ed.), *Fractures of the Tibia: A Clinical Casebook*,
DOI 10.1007/978-3-319-21774-1_9

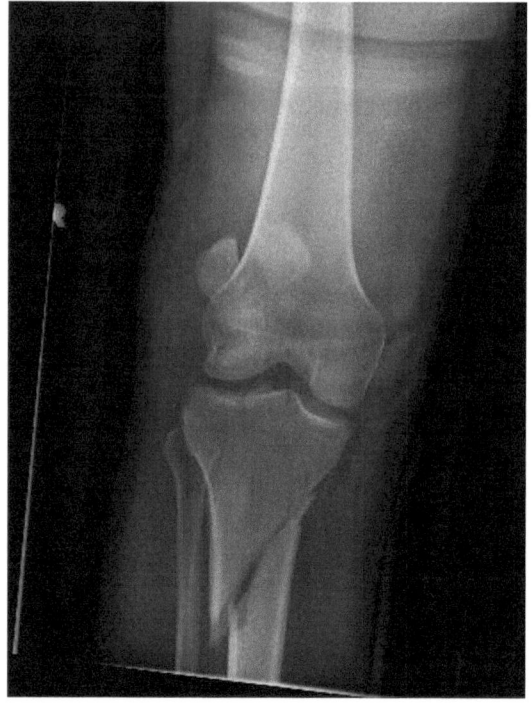

Fig. 9.1 AP X-ray view of right knee demonstrating a proximal tibia fracture and patella fracture

Treatment and Timing of Surgery

Decision was made to treat this fracture with plate and screw fixation to avoid additional insult to the extensor mechanism, and also to not risk displacement of the intraarticular extension. The significant soft tissue swelling and contusion precluded early ORIF. An external fixator was placed initially to manage the soft tissues. Definitive ORIF was performed 13 days post injury.

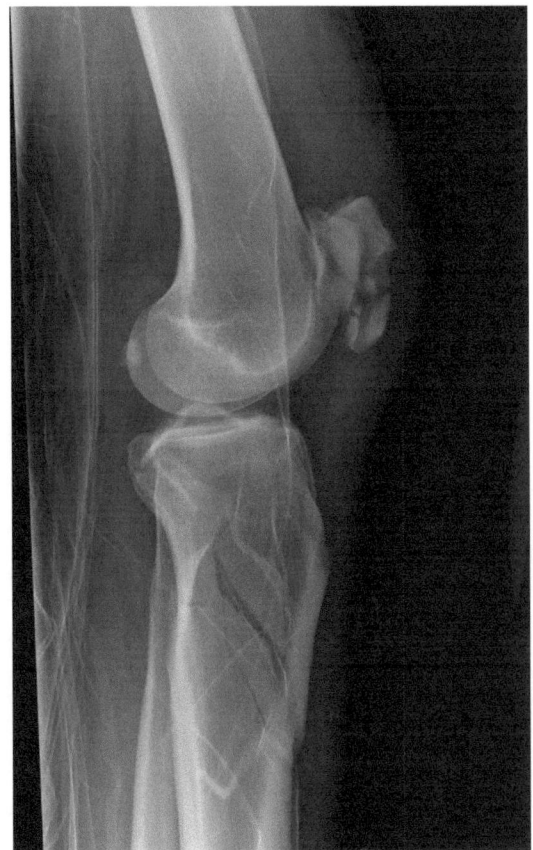

Fig. 9.2 Lateral X-ray view of right knee demonstrating a proximal tibia fracture and patella fracture

Surgical Tact

Position

Supine, with a small bump under knee, which maintained acceptable fracture alignment in the sagittal plane.

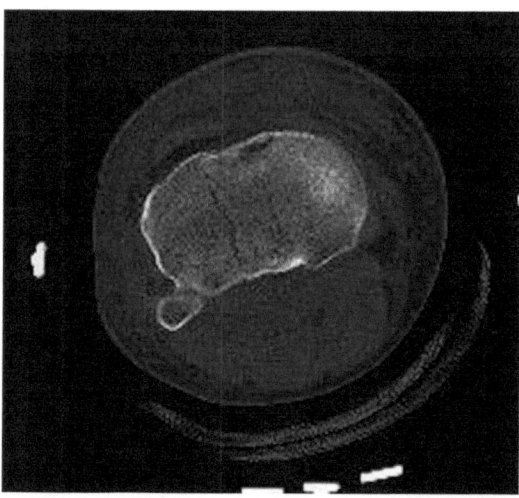

Fig. 9.3 Axial CT scan image demonstrating 2 undisplaced fracture lines at the level of the tibial plateau

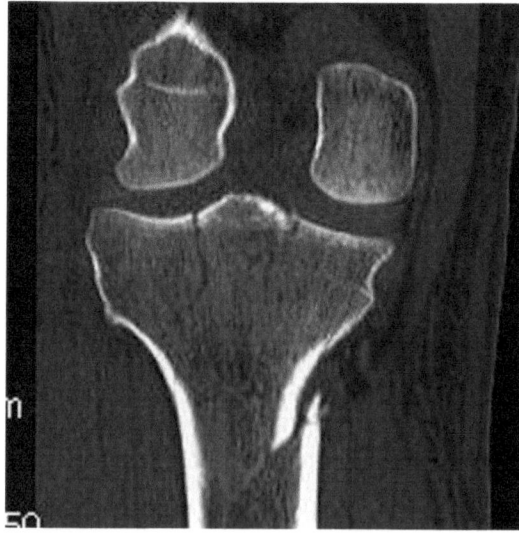

Fig. 9.4 Coronal CT scan image demonstrating extension of the proximal tibia fracture into the tibial plateau

Approach

Minimally invasive plate osteosynthesis, using lateral and medial incisions over the proximal, middle, and distal tibia.

Fracture Reduction

A periarticular clamp was applied through stab incisions to maintain reduction of the undisplaced intraarticular fracture lines. A lateral approach to the proximal tibia was done using a curvilinear incision from the lateral condyle to Gerdy's tubercle. Exposure of the proximal lateral surface of the tibia with elevation of the anterior compartment was performed. Two 6.5 mm cannulated cancellous screws were inserted – one from medial to lateral and the second from lateral to medial. This configuration left ample room for plate placement laterally while providing stable fixation across the articular surface. The periarticular clamp was removed (Figs. 9.5 and 9.6).

A targeted locking plate was slid submuscularly underneath the anterior compartment and positioned on the proximal tibial fragment under direct visualization and under fluoroscopy. Periarticular clamps were used to reduce the plate to the bone proximally, and unicortical locking screws were inserted (Fig. 9.7).

A pulling device ("Whirlybird") was used to reduce the distal fragment toward the plate and align the fracture in the coronal and sagittal planes (Figs. 9.8 and 9.9). Locking screws were inserted distally to maintain reduction and alignment.

A reconstruction plate was contoured to fit the medial tibia and slid anterograde through a small proximal medial incision. A second small incision was made at the distal end of the medial plate. The plate was reduced to the tibia using small periarticular clamps and secured to the proximal tibia with locking screws. Cortical screws were then inserted distally, the first in buttress mode, to complete the fixation and resist any varus collapse (Figs. 9.10 and 9.11).

Final images demonstrate anatomic alignment and stable fixation (Figs. 9.12 and 9.13). Skin staples illustrate the placement of multiple small incisions.

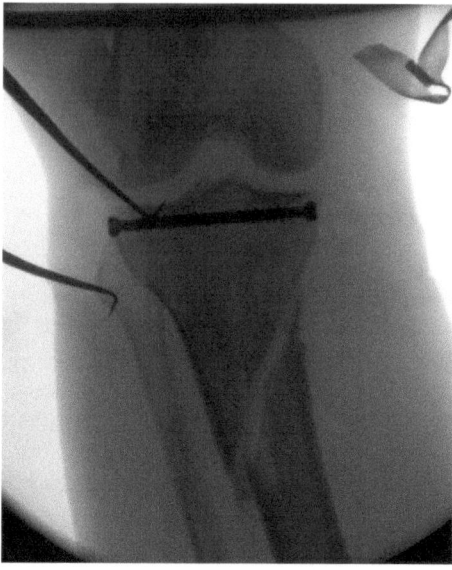

Fig. 9.5 Intra-operative AP view of the proximal tibia with medial and lateral
screw placement

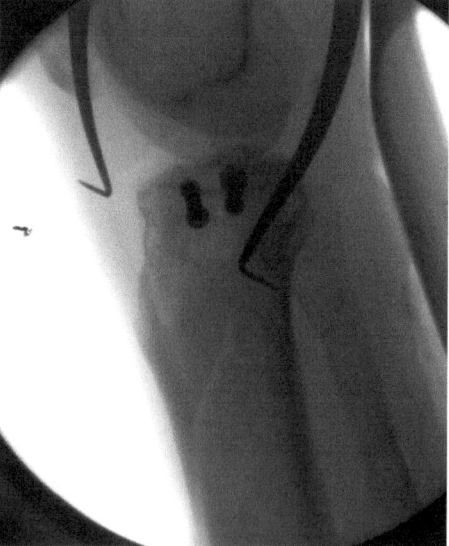

Fig. 9.6 Intra-operative Lateral view of the proximal tibia with medial and
lateral screw placement

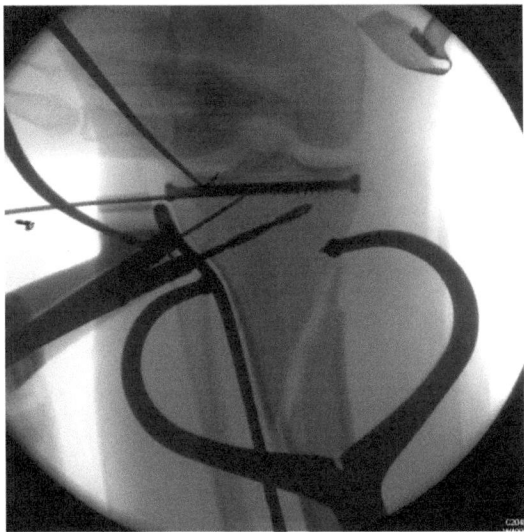

Fig. 9.7 Intra-operative AP view of the proximal tibia demonstrating plate reduction and proximal fixation

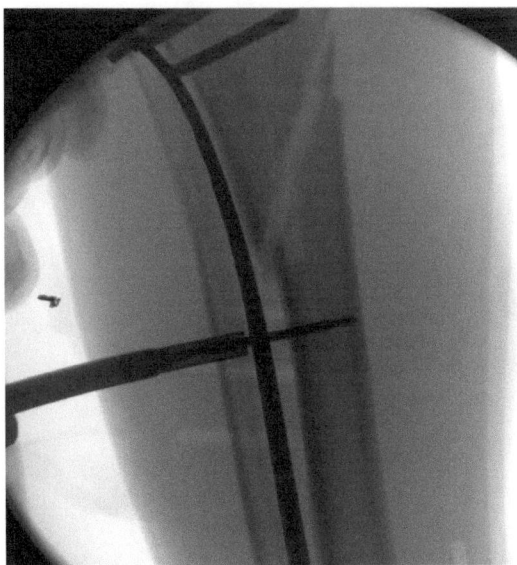

Fig. 9.8 Intra-operative AP view of the tibia demonstrating application of the "Whirlybird" to correct translation in the coronal plane

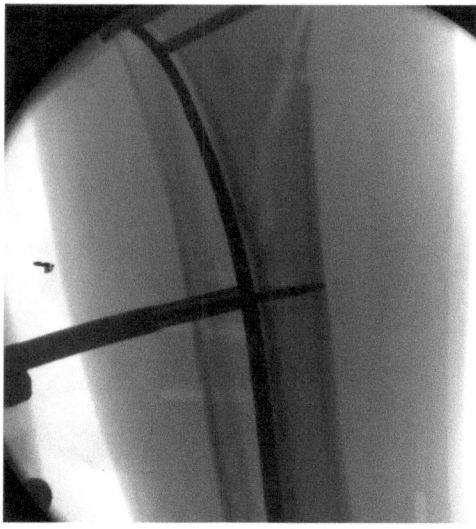

Fig. 9.9 Intra-operative AP view of the tibia after correction of translation in the coronal plane

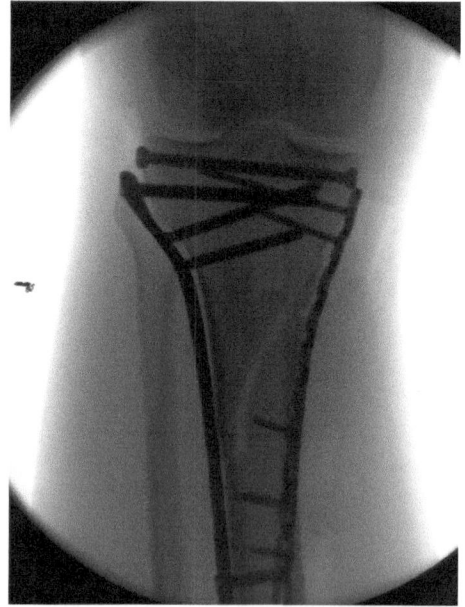

Fig. 9.10 Intra-operative AP view of the tibia with medial fixation

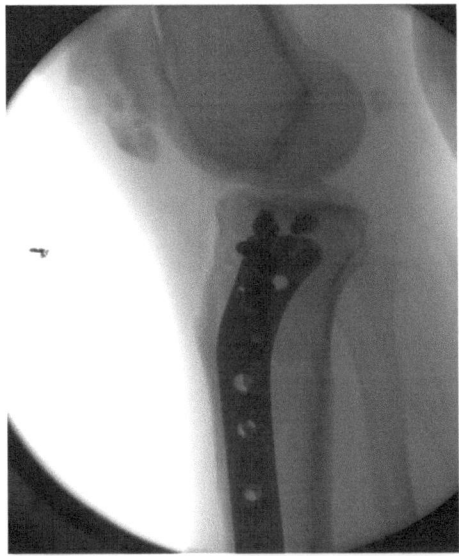

Fig. 9.11 Intra-operative Lateral view of the tibia after medial fixation

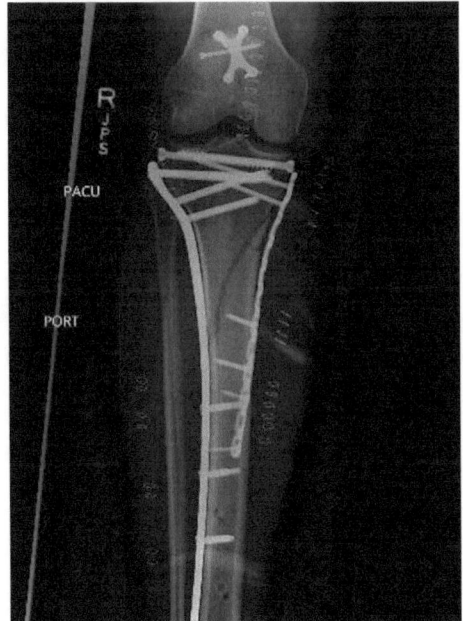

Fig. 9.12 Post-operative AP X-ray view of the tibia

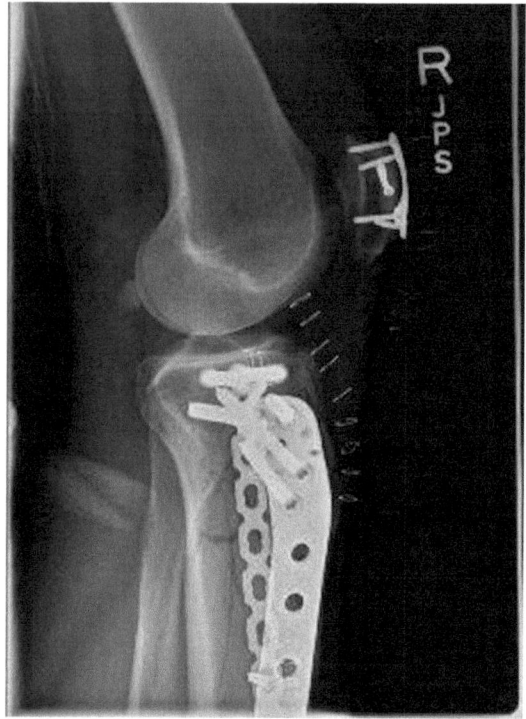

Fig. 9.13 Post-operative Lateral X-ray view of the proximal tibia

Postoperative Plan

Soft dressing and knee immobilizer were applied for comfort
and for nighttime wear. He was referred to therapy for knee and
ankle range of motion, non-weight-bearing for 12 weeks. Knee
ROM was limited to active flexion and passive extension in the
prone position, secondary to the patella fracture. Clinical and
radiographic follow-ups were done till union.

Outcome

Follow-up radiographs at 8 months show healed fracture (Figs. 9.14 and 9.15). Patient complained of pain over the proximal lateral hardware, no extensor lag, and knee flexion to 95°. He returned to the operating room at 9 months post operation for removal of hardware and manipulation under anesthesia. At 1 year postoperatively, he had full extension with no extensor lag, and 130° of knee flexion. No complaints of knee pain and no limitations related to the right knee injury.

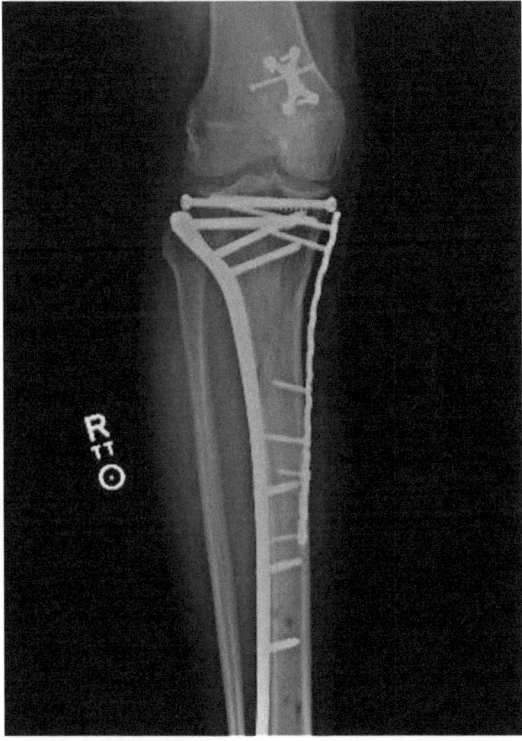

Fig. 9.14 AP X-ray view of the tibia at 8 months post-operative demonstrating successful union of the tibia fracture

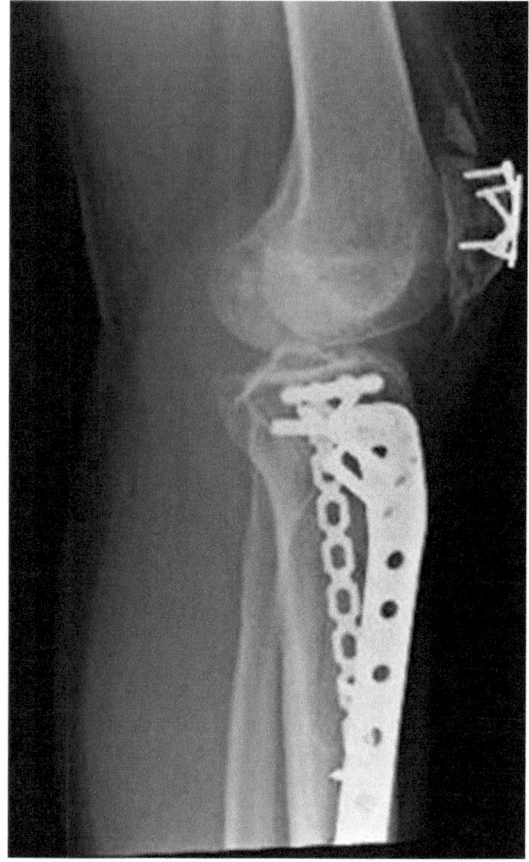

Fig. 9.15 Lateral X-ray view of the tibia at 8 months post-operative demonstrating successful union of the tibia fracture

Complications

Symptomatic hardware, loss of knee flexion.

Salient Points/Pearls

- Careful soft tissue management is essential in order to avoid wound complications and minimize infection.

- When necessary, external fixation is used to maintain overall length and alignment while waiting for the swelling to decrease and soft tissue contusion to resolve.
- When possible, external fixation pin placement should be outside of the planned area for definitive plate placement.
- If external fixation is used for longer than approximately 2 weeks, or pin sites become infected, a "pin holiday" should be used to try to minimize infection. Either the external fixator is removed and a splint is applied, or the pin locations are changed.
- If fasciotomy wounds are present, the risk of infection with the use of surface implants such as plates and screws increases significantly, and intramedullary nailing should be considered.
- If the fracture site is exposed, a small 2.7 or 3.5 mm plate with unicortical screws can be used to maintain provisional anatomic alignment.
- Isolated lateral locking plate placement may be adequate for the management of low-energy proximal tibial fractures, especially in patients who are able to reliably maintain their NWB status and those without significant medial comminution.
- If distal lateral screw placement is necessary – typically past the 10th or 11th hole on a proximal tibial locking plate – a more generous distal incision with careful dissection should be used to avoid an iatrogenic injury to the superficial peroneal nerve with distal screw placement.

Suggested Reading

Ruffolo MR, Gettys FK, Montijo HE, Seymour RB, Karunakar MA. Complications of high-energy bicondylar tibial plateau fractures treated with dual plating through two incisions. J Orthop Trauma. 2015;29(2):85–90.

Shah CM, Babb PE, McAndrew CM, Brimmo O, Badarudeen S, Tornetta III P, Ricci WM, Gardner MJ. Definitive plates overlapping provisional external fixator pin sites: is the infection risk increased? J Orthop Trauma. 2014;28(9):518–22.

Lee SM, Oh CW, Oh JK, Kim JW, Lee HJ, Chon CS, Lee BJ, Kyung HS. Biomechanical analysis of operative methods in the treatment of extraarticular fracture of the proximal tibia. Clin Orthop Surg. 2014;6(3):312–7.

Phisitkul P, Mckinley TO, Nepola JV, Marsh JL. Complications of locking plate fixation in complex proximal tibia injuries. J Orthop Trauma. 2007;21(2):83–91.

Deangelis JP, Deangelis NA, Anderson R. Anatomy of the superficial peroneal nerve in relation to fixation of tibia fractures with the less invasive stabilization system. J Orthop Trauma. 2004;18(8):536–9.

Chapter 10
Mid Shaft Tibia Shaft Fracture Treated with Intra-medullary Nail (IMN)

Lisa K. Cannada

Case Presentation

A 29-year-old male presented with a midshaft tibial fracture after a motorcycle accident. He had an isolated, closed midshaft tibial fracture. There was clinical evaluation for compartment syndrome, and his pulses were well felt with no neurological injury. A long leg splint was applied.

Injury Films

Injury films (AP and lateral) demonstrate a midshaft tibial fracture with comminution (Fig. 10.1).

L.K. Cannada, MD
Division of Orthopaedic Surgery, Saint Louis University,
St. Louis, MD, USA
e-mail: lcannada@slu.edu

© Springer International Publishing Switzerland 2016   121
N.C. Tejwani (ed.), *Fractures of the Tibia: A Clinical Casebook*,
DOI 10.1007/978-3-319-21774-1_10

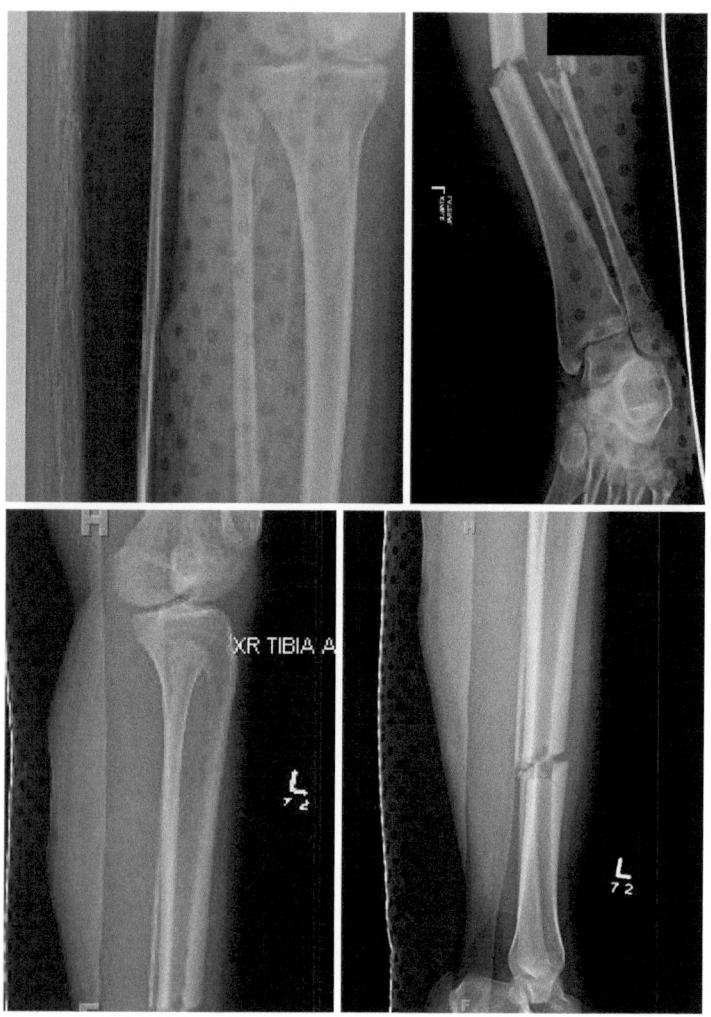

Fig. 10.1

Radiographs Needed

1. Injury films: AP/lateral of tibia to include knee and ankle joint. As demonstrated with this case, oftentimes there are more than one X-ray for each view. Be sure to evaluate carefully, as initial radiographs may be taken with field splints in place and may obscure fracture details. Postreduction radiographs often are in a splint, again obscuring details. Scrutinize carefully each fracture for additional injuries!
2. Intraop fluoroscopy for starting point; reduction; initial reaming and nail placement.
3. Postop films
4. Follow-up radiographs until demonstration of union

Treatment and Timing of Surgery

This case presented to the emergency room in the late evening hours. Clinical exam was completed overnight and documented every 2–3 h to rule out compartment syndrome [1]. The patient was scheduled for the trauma room as first case the next morning. A detailed discussion about the options for nonoperative treatment with casting versus nailing was had, and a decision to proceed with IMN was made [2].

Surgical Tact

Position

Supine, with bump (triangle) under knee

Approach

Midline incision with patella tendon split in line with its fibers and approach to proximal starting point, as seen on fluoroscopy views (Fig. 10.2). When obtaining your fluoroscopy images, be sure to obtain true AP and lateral images, so that your starting point is correct.

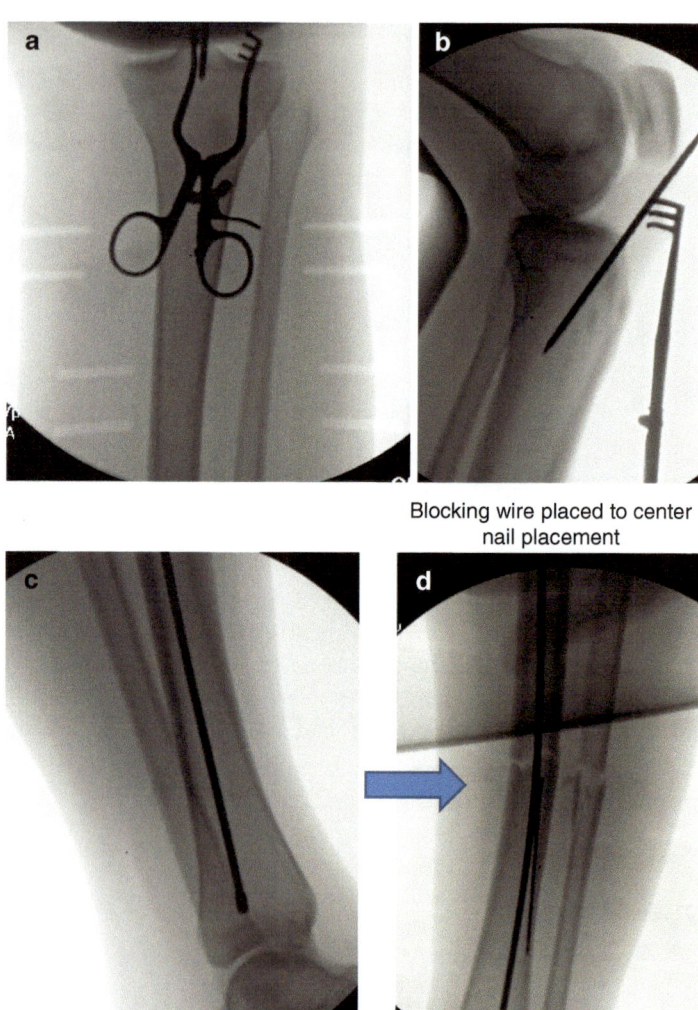

Blocking wire placed to center
nail placement

Fig. 10.2

Fracture Reduction

Fracture was reduced using manual traction or can be reduced with an external fixator (pins in calcaneus and posterior proximal tibia). A small blocking wire was inserted to center the nail (Fig. 10.3).

To determine the desired nail diameter, once chatter is encountered, we over ream by 1.0 to 1.5 mm. Two locking screws were used at the proximal end in static mode. Distally, two medial to lateral screws were used after obtaining perfect circles and placing the interlocking screws using freehand technique (Fig. 10.4).

Final radiographs demonstrated fracture reduced with IMN in place (Fig. 10.5).

Blocking wire

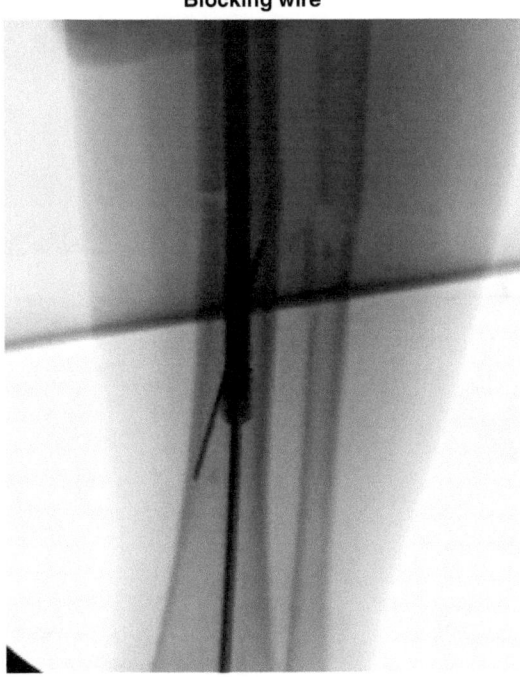

Fig. 10.3

Fig. 10.4

Tip: Use two drill bits to make it easier for trajectory when placing interlocking screws

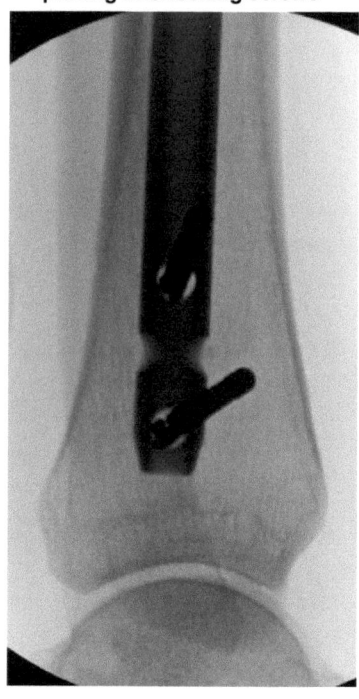

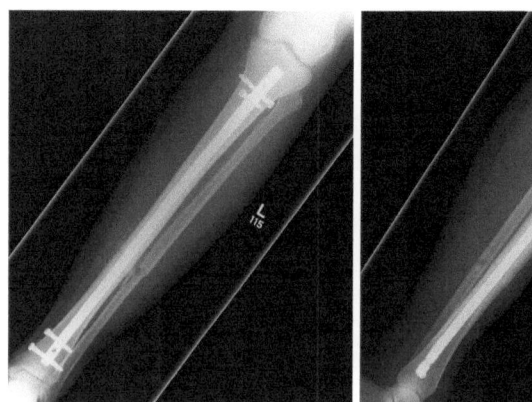
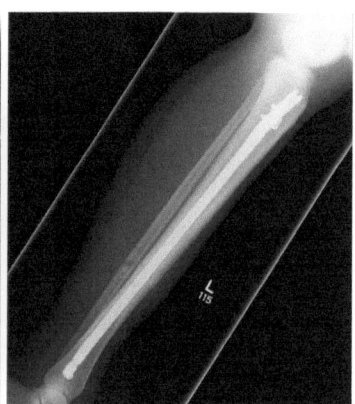

Fig. 10.5

Postoperative Plan

A short leg splint was placed initially, and then prior to discharge, patient was placed in a CAM boot. Due to fracture comminution, the patient was made partial weight-bearing. He was referred to therapy for knee and ankle range of motion as well. Clinical and radiographic follow-up was completed until fracture united.

Outcome

Follow-up radiographs at 6 months demonstrate healed fracture. He has resumed motorcycle riding.

Complications

None.

Salient Points/Pearls

- The starting point may be obtained through a medial parapatellar, a patellar splitting, or some surgeons prefer to use a suprapatellar technique, depending on the fracture pattern and preference [3]. There are special instruments to protect the patella and knee with suprapatellar nailing.
- Fracture reduction can be achieved through temporary external fixation/travel traction (Fig. 10.6), manual manipulation, and percutaneous well-placed clamps or small plates. In addition, in some instances, a small incision may be used for open reduction of difficult fractures. This chapter demonstrated use of a blocking Kirschner wire to assist in reduction and nail placement. The diaphysis is a smaller region than the metaphysis; so, these wires may be useful if carefully placed. In fractures involving the metaphyseal region, blocking screws may be used to guide the nail and assist in the reduction of the fracture [4].

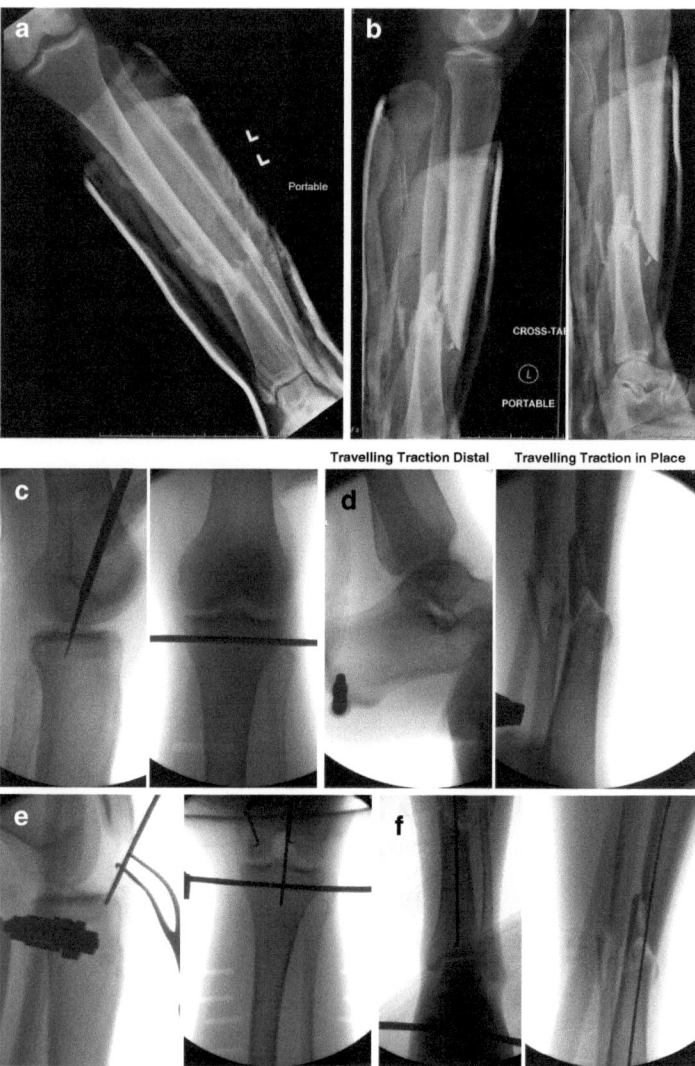

Fig. 10.6 Case Example, (**a**) Pre-Op AP, (**b**) Pre-Op Lateral, (**c**) Inserting Travelling Traction Proximal, (**d**) Before We Start, (**e**) Getting Starting Point, (**f**) Guide wire Placement, (**g**) Intra-op Tips, (**h**) Perfect Circles for Interlocking, (**i**) Ap Post Op, (**j**) Lateral Post Op.

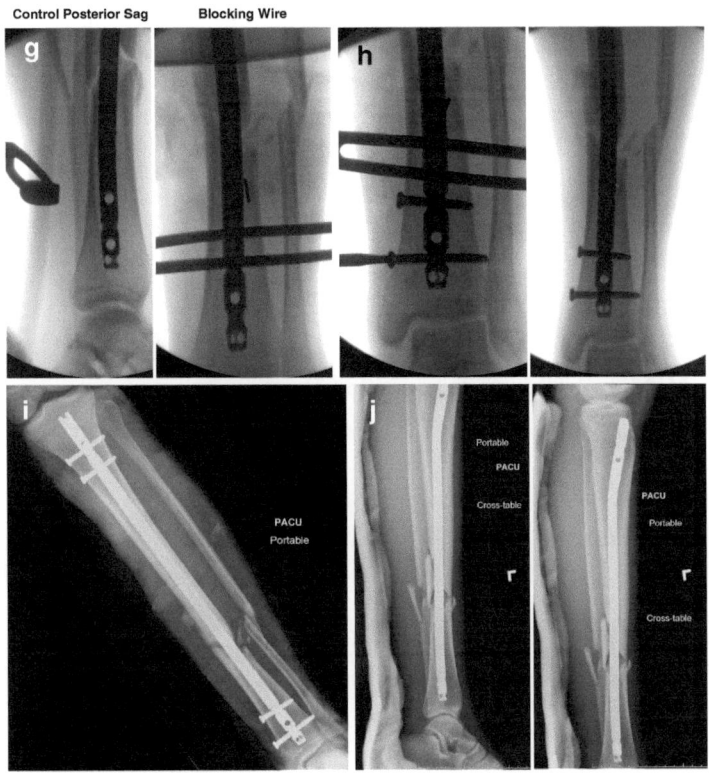

Fig. 10.6 (continued)

- Two proximal and two distal static locking screws are recommended.
- Postoperatively, weight-bearing of midshaft tibial fractures is dependent upon fracture pattern and bone loss. There is limited soft tissue medially, and high-energy injuries may have a poor soft tissue envelope, as seen in closed fractures.
- High-energy tibial shaft fractures should all be evaluated for compartment syndrome. Compartment syndrome is a clinical diagnosis; so, in awake and alert patients, serial clinical exams are helpful. For those patients who are obtunded or cannot cooperate, compartment syndrome needs to be ruled out [1].

- Complications may include infection, delayed union, or non-union. In addition, the patients should be counseled regarding knee pain from nail insertion, which resolves over time [5]. There may be painful hardware from prominent interlocking screws. Close attention to detail with insertion can be helpful.

Mid Shaft Tibia

The Starting Point
Make sure guidewire centered on both views

Mid Shaft Tibia with Travelling Traction

Pre-Op AP

References

1. Taylor RM, Sullivan MP, Mehta S. Acute compartment syndrome: obtaining diagnosis, providing treatment, and minimizing medicolegal risk. Curr Rev Musculoskelet Med. 2012;5(3):206–13. doi:10.1007/s12178-012-9126-y.
2. Duan X, Al-Qwbani M, Zeng Y, Zhang W, Xiang Z. Intramedullary nailing for tibial shaft fractures in adults. Cochrane Database Syst Rev. 2012;1:CD008241. doi:10.1002/14651858.CD008241.pub2. Review.
3. Gelbke MK, Coombs D, Powell S, DiPasquale TG. Suprapatellar versus infra-patellar intramedullary nail insertion of the tibia: a cadaveric model for comparison of patellofemoral contact pressures and forces. J Orthop Trauma. 2010;24(11):665–71. doi:10.1097/BOT.0b013e3181f6c001.
4. Schemitsch EH, Bhandari M, Guyatt G, Sanders DW, Swiontkowski M, Tornetta P, Walter SD, Zdero R, Goslings JC, Teague D, Jeray K, McKee MD, Study to Prospectively Evaluate Reamed Intramedullary Nails in Patients with Tibial Fractures (SPRINT) Investigators. Prognostic factors for predicting outcomes after intramedullary nailing of the tibia. J Bone Joint Surg Am. 2012;94(19):1786–93. doi:10.2106/JBJS.J.01418.
5. Väistö O, Toivanen J, Kannus P, Järvinen M. Anterior knee pain after intramedullary nailing of fractures of the tibial shaft: an eight-year follow-up of a prospective, randomized study comparing two different nail-insertion techniques. J Trauma. 2008;64(6):1511–6. doi:10.1097/TA.0b013e318031cd27.

Chapter 11
Tibia Shaft Distal Third: Treatment with an Intramedullary Nail

Juan Favela and Cory A. Collinge

Background

The use of statically locked, reamed intramedullary nails has become the standard of care for the vast majority of tibial shaft fractures in adults [1, 2]. The restoration of relatively normal anatomy (length, angular, and rotational) is a standard goal of tibial nailing, and if not accomplished or if the leg falls into malalignment postoperatively, chronic pain, arthrosis, gait abnormalities, and other problems may

The authors have received nothing of value relating to their preparation of this manuscript.

Conflicts of Interest   Dr. Collinge has a royalty agreement with Biomet Orthopedics; Mr. Favela has no conflict to report.

J. Favela, BS
Harvard University, Boston, MA, USA

Orthopedic Specialty Associates, Fort Worth, TX 76104, USA
e-mail: Jfavela1192@gmail.com

C.A. Collinge, MD (✉)
Orthopedic Trauma, Harris Methodist Fort Worth Hospital/John Peter Smith Orthopedic Surgery Residency,
800 5th Ave., Suite 500, Fort Worth, TX 76104, USA
e-mail: ccollinge@msn.com

© Springer International Publishing Switzerland 2016   131
N.C. Tejwani (ed.), *Fractures of the Tibia: A Clinical Casebook*,
DOI 10.1007/978-3-319-21774-1_11

ensue over time [3, 4]. Due to cortical thinning and medullary cavity expansion present at the metadiaphyseal areas of the tibia, distal third fractures are at risk of malalignment during nailing and often require additional steps to ensure a high-quality reduction and adequate stability. Unlike isthmal fractures, the intramedullary nail itself does not assist with reduction of distal shaft fracture patterns, although it still maintains a level of biomechanical stability and axial support that still makes it the treatment of choice for these injuries.

Optimally, prior to the insertion of an intramedullary nail, one should establish appropriate alignment and rotation of the fractured bone. This can be done via a number of methods: manual manipulation, use of femoral/universal distractor, fibular plating, Steinmann pin or Schanz screw joysticks, unicortical plating, pointed reduction clamping, blocking screws, or others. It is important to note that provisional reduction should be maintained during all instrumentation for nailing: guide wire insertion, reaming, nail insertion, and interlocking.

Short Clinical History/Scenario

We present the case example of an active, 33-year-old man who suffered injury to the right leg as a result of jumping down from a 6 ft fence. He was previously healthy, and no other injuries were identified in his evaluation for this injury. He was splinted in the emergency department and admitted to the hospital.

Treatment Considerations/Planning/Tests Needed

The pattern of injury, site, and patient factors were considered. The injury was not "high-energy" by mechanism (moderate) or injury pattern (closed fracture, simple pattern). Compartment syndrome did not appear to be present and there was a normal neurovascular examination. Plain AP and lateral radiographs showed a spiral fracture of the distal third tibial shaft and associated fibula fracture (Fig. 11.1). No advanced imaging appeared indicated in this case, although additional studies are often helpful in patients with tibial shaft fractures. A trauma evaluation including ATLS

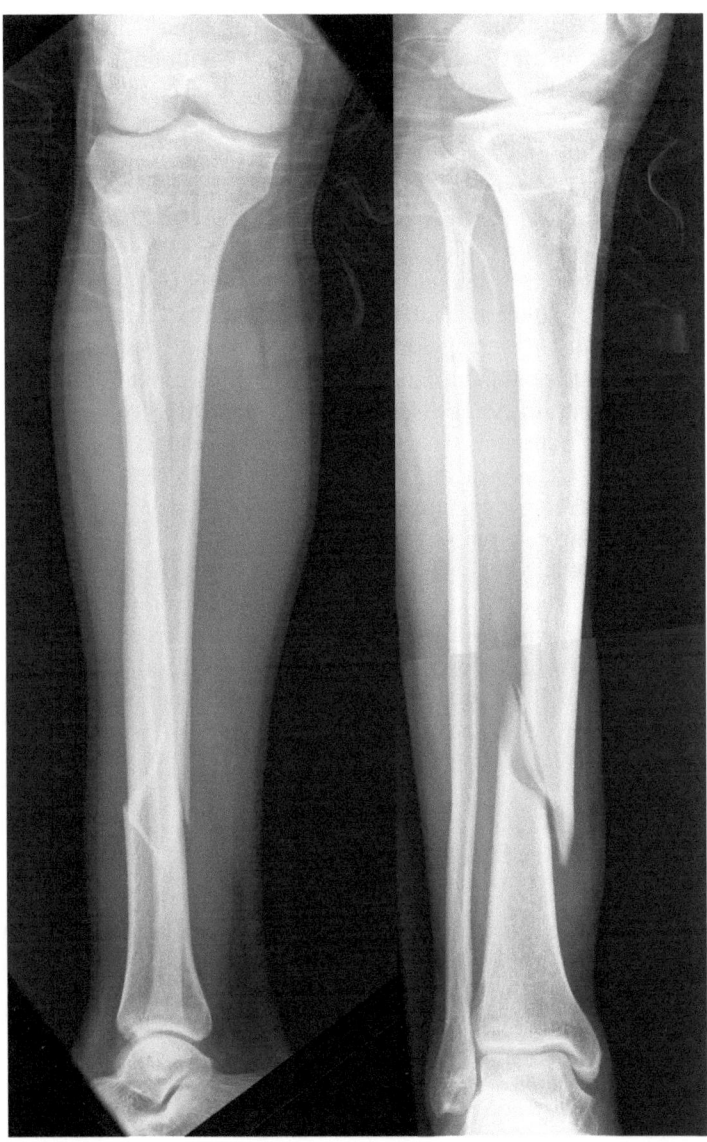

Fig. 11.1 Anteroposterior and lateral plain radiographs of the leg of a 33-year-old man with distal third spiral fracture of the tibia and associated fibula fracture

protocols must be initiated for high-energy mechanisms: other traumatic injuries are commonly associated with tibial shaft fractures in that setting. Dedicated plain X-rays or computed tomography of the ankle is helpful if there are any radiographic abnormalities of the articular distal tibia. Posterior malleolus fractures are found in 25 % of patients with selected tibial fractures, and spiral fractures of the distal third are probably the most likely shaft pattern to be associated with ankle injury [5].

Casting or cast-bracing was at one time the standard of care for this injury pattern and still has excellent utility in treating pediatric patients: problems with malunion, ankle stiffness, and patient tolerance are common in adults [1, 6]. Plating remains an option in tibial shaft fractures associated with far proximal or distal tibial fractures where limited fixation with a nail would be expected [7]. That said, techniques and nails have evolved in the past decade, which have widely expanded the indications for nailing. Temporizing external fixation is often indicated in the polytrauma patient or one with a high-energy open tibial fracture where damage control measures are indicated. Second, in complex fractures such as one with soft tissue problems or even infection, circular frame external fixation may be successfully utilized [7].

In the case presented previously, treatment options were discussed with the patient, and he opted for treatment with intramedullary tibial nailing.

Timing of Surgery

As there were no factors complicating treatment, the patient underwent closed, reamed intramedullary nailing of the tibia, the morning after injury.

Intraoperative Tips and Tricks for Reduction/ Fixation

The patient was taken to the operating room and given general anesthesia. He was then positioned on the radiolucent operating table in the supine position. All bony prominences and pressure points were well padded. A paralytic agent was given to allow the surgeons to successfully manipulate the fracture into gross position (including regaining length). A wide, thorough, sterile orthopedic prep of the entire right lower extremity was performed. Preoperative antibiotics were administered.

Setup includes the leg supported on a size-appropriate radiolucent triangle and the C-arm brought in from the contralateral side.

The first portion of the case required gaining a quality reduction. We prefer obtaining the reduction and holding it passively with surgical instruments instead of using manual techniques throughout the case. The advantages of this approach are less demand for surgical assistance, reliable maintenance of reduction (does not get tired), and no ill effect to the object holding reduction from radiation exposure. Specifically, -the standard reduction for simple spiral or oblique tibial shaft fractures uses manual traction to restore gross alignment (Fig. 11.2), and then percutaneous application of a large pointed clamp to finalize the reduction and maintain it for the remainder of the nailing (Fig. 11.3) [8] We use a modified pointed clamp that allows for wider excursion than a standard Weber clamp, which may prevent impinging on the soft tissues. Small stab incisions are made, allowing for the clamp's tines to be placed (Fig. 11.2). Usually one tine is placed posterolaterally and the other anteromedially, but placement must be confirmed via the C-arm. For truly transverse fractures below the isthmus (rare), manipulation into position will create a relatively stable reduction for nailing. In comminuted fracture patterns, we prefer to use a femoral distractor (or even two) to regain length and alignment during nailing.

The second portion of the procedure was access to the proximal tibia. A 1-in. incision was made over the medial aspect of the patellar ligament, and a sharp awl was placed on the appropriate entry portal for insertion of the tibial nail. This was confirmed on multiple C-arm views. Access to the intramedullary canal was then gained. The ball-tip guide wire was passed to the level of the fracture. Indirect reduction was then achieved using pointed reduction clamps, and the wire passed across the fracture and into the distal segment, where it was tapped into the bone just above the ankle.

Light sequential reaming was then performed with bullet-tip deep fluted reamers until chatter was encountered (12 mm). The reduction was maintained during reaming, nail insertion, and

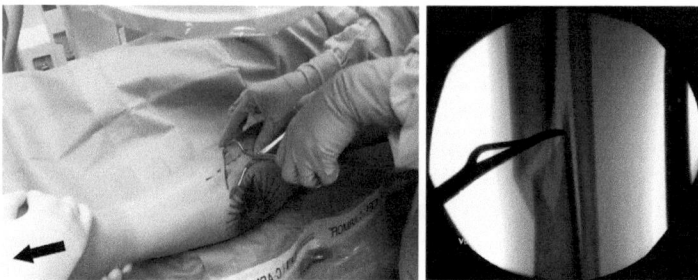

Fig. 11.2 Clinical picture showing that stab incisions are planned for clamp placement and that gross length and rotation have been restored by simple traction (*black arrow*). Corresponding C-arm image is also shown

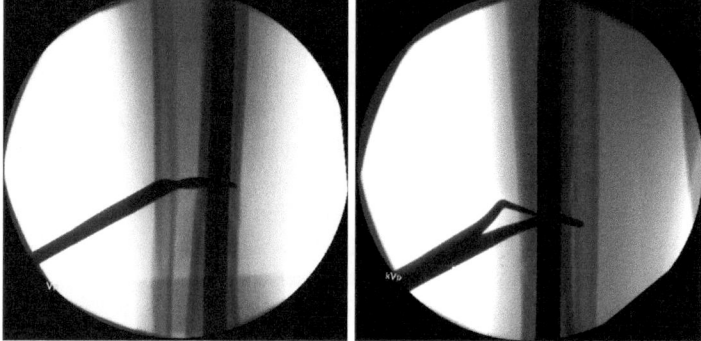

Fig. 11.3 Radiographic images with the clamp applied holding quality reduction for the remainder of the case

locking. A 10.5 × 350 mm nail was inserted over the guide wire and tapped to the appropriate depth. The guide wire was then removed. Two distal locking screws were then applied using a freehand technique. A proximal locking screw was placed using the jig system. The insertion device was then removed, and the knee joint was irrigated with copious amounts of saline and suctioned repeatedly to remove the reamings. The reduction clamp was then removed. Final C-arm images were obtained, which confirmed the appropriateness of alignment and implants (Fig. 11.4). The knee wound was closed in a multilayer fashion. The locking screw sites were closed in a simple fashion.

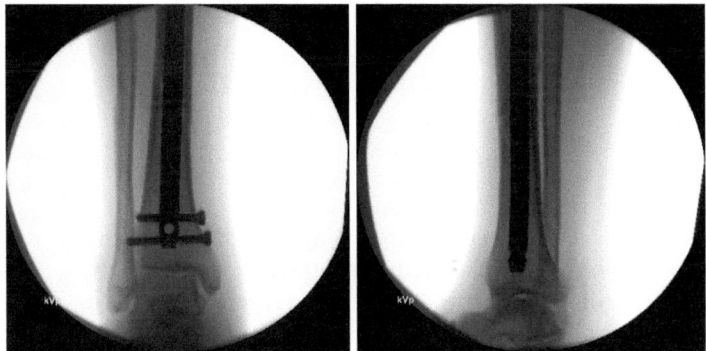

Fig. 11.4 Postnailing C-arm images showing improved alignment and appropriate implants

The patient tolerated these procedures well and postoperatively was extubated and taken to the recovery room.

Postoperative Protocols Including Splint/Cast and Timing of Weight-Bearing

Postoperatively, the patient was transferred back to the orthopedic floor for elevation, pain control, and monitoring. He was seen by physical therapy and mobilized reasonably well over the next 24 h. Weight-bearing status of the patient after surgery was 20-lb limit on the injured leg wearing a boot. His pain was well controlled first on intravenous and then oral pain medication. His wounds were stable at the time of his discharge on postoperative day 1. His hospital course was otherwise uncomplicated.

Follow-Up with Union/Complications

Follow-up included a 7–10 day office visit for suture removal. Emphasis was placed on swelling control and range of motion at the knee and ankle. In contrast to stable isthmal fractures, we authors prefer to keep patients with spiral, long oblique, or highly comminuted distal third tibial fractures protected weight-bearing in the early postoperative period, for example, the first 6 weeks.

No complications were seen in this case.

Salient Points/Pearls

- Evaluate all tibia fractures with high-energy mechanism for possible open injury and compartment syndrome.
- Identifying intraarticular extension is important before starting surgery and may need CT scans.
- Reduction of the fracture before reaming is useful for appropriate nail placement and alignment.
- Use of biologically friendly bone-reduction clamps will allow reduction being held more reliably with minimum radiation to the surgeon's or assistant's hands.
- Tibial shaft fractures are relatively slow to heal. One might estimate this fracture to be completely healed at 4–5 months.

References

1. Karladani AH, et al. Displaced tibial shaft fractures: a prospective randomized study of closed intramedullary nailing versus cast treatment in 53 patients. Acta Orthop. 2000;71(2):160–7.
2. Finkemeier CG, Schmidt AH, Kyle RF, Templeman DC, Varecka TF. A prospective, randomized study of intramedullary nails inserted with and without reaming for the treatment of open and closed fractures of the tibial shaft. J Orthop Trauma. 2000;14(3):187–93.
3. Puno RM, Vaughan JJ, Stetten ML, Johnson JR. Long-term effects of tibial angular malunion on the knee and ankle joints. J Orthop Trauma. 1991;5(3):247–54.
4. Milner SA, Davis TRC, Muir KR, Greenwood DC, Doherty M. Long-term outcome after tibial shaft fracture: is malunion important? J Bone Joint Surg. 2002;84(6):971–80.
5. Kukkonen J, Heikkilä JT, Kyyrönen T, Mattila K, Gullichsen E. Posterior malleolar fracture is often associated with spiral tibial diaphyseal fracture: a retrospective study. J Trauma Acute Care Surg. 2006;60(5):1058–60.
6. Bone LB, Sucato D, Stegemann PM, Rohrbacher BJ. Displaced isolated fractures of the tibial shaft treated with either a cast or intramedullary nailing. An outcome analysis of matched pairs of patients*. J Bone Joint Surg. 1997;79(9):1336–41.

7. Zelle BA, Bhandari M, Espiritu M, Koval KJ, Zlowodzki M, Evidence-Based Orthopaedic Trauma Working Group. Treatment of distal tibia fractures without articular involvement: a systematic review of 1125 fractures. J Orthop Trauma. 2006;20(1):76–9.

8. Collinge CA, Beltran M. Percutaneous clamping of spiral and oblique fractures of the tibial shaft: a safe and effective reduction Aid during intramedullary nailing percutaneous clamping of spiral and oblique fractures of the tibial shaft: a safe and effective reduction aid during intramedullary nailing. J Orthop Trauma. 2015;29(6):e208–12.

Chapter 12
Distal Tibia Shaft Fracture Treated with Plate Fixation

Chase C. Woodward and Jaimo Ahn

Case Presentation

A 33-year-old woman who denied past medical history was brought to the trauma bay by ambulance with left leg pain after being struck while on her bicycle by an automobile. She had deep wounds on her left posterior calf and medial ankle. She was neurovascularly intact (motor and sensory) to the left distal extremity with minimal-to-moderate swelling and soft compartments to palpation. Radiographs demonstrated left distal tibial shaft and tibial plateau fractures. The only other injury was a superficial abrasion to her chin. She was cooperative with the exam and hemodynamically stable. No other major injuries were identified.

Injury Films

AP and lateral radiographs of the left ankle and tibia/fibula demonstrated a mildly displaced distal third tibial shaft spiral fracture with subcutaneous air indicating an open injury. There was no

C.C. Woodward, MD, MPH • J. Ahn, MD, PhD, FACS (✉)
Department of Orthopaedic Surgery, University of Pennsylvania,
Philadelphia, PA, USA
e-mail: jaimo_ahn@alumni.stanford.edu

© Springer International Publishing Switzerland 2016   141
N.C. Tejwani (ed.), *Fractures of the Tibia: A Clinical Casebook*,
DOI 10.1007/978-3-319-21774-1_12

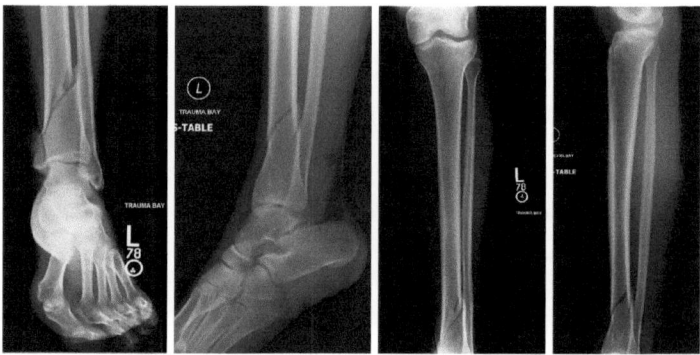

Fig. 12.1 AP and lateral radiographs of the left ankle and tibia/fibula

definite evidence of fracture extension into the ankle articular surface. There was also a lucent line through the proximal tibia representing a lateral tibial plateau fracture. The fibula was intact. No CT scan was performed at the time of initial evaluation (Fig. 12.1).

Treatment and Timing of Surgery

This tibial shaft fracture was treated as an open injury. The patient was expeditiously administered intravenous cefazolin and genta- micin. The open wounds were irrigated at the bedside and sterile dressings applied. Subsequently, the left leg was placed in a long leg plaster splint. The patient provided informed consent for urgent debridement and fixation of the open fracture site. The need to go to the operating room for emergent debridement is debatable, and recent literature suggests that delay up to 8–12 h if medically indicated may not alter the outcomes as long as antibiot- ics were administered expeditiously.

There was discussion among the orthopedic team regarding the appropriateness of external fixation of the distal tibial fracture versus acute definitive fixation. Because there was no gross con- tamination, minimal swelling, and concomitant ipsilateral tibial plateau injury, acute definitive open reduction and plate fixation following debridement and irrigation was planned. In terms of fixation strategy, the long oblique nature of the fracture with minimal comminution made the injury amenable to the application of interfragmentary compression and spanning plate utilizing absolute stability principles.

Surgical Tact

Position

Supine on a regular operating room table (with optional distal extension for ease of fluoroscopy maneuvering), operative leg on a radiolucent foam ramp, a rolled blanket bump under ipsilateral hip, and fluoroscopy machine from the contralateral side of the table.

Approach

Initially, the open wounds were extended and thoroughly debrided and irrigated with 6 L of saline. Subsequently, the tibial shaft fracture was percutaneously reduced and initially fixed with a cortical screw. Finally, a medial ankle incision was used to insert a precontoured plate in a minimally invasive fashion.

Fracture Reduction and Fixation

Following open wound debridement, stab incisions were made on the medial and lateral sides of the tibia at the level of the fracture (fluoroscopically guided; see images) for the percutaneous insertion of a point-to-point reduction clamp. The intact fibula was helpful in gauging the proper tibial length during reduction. With gentle manipulation of the distal extremity and careful application of the clamp tongs, appropriate reduction and compression was achieved and confirmed on fluoroscopic imaging. The oblique nature of the fracture made it amenable to fixation with a 3.5 mm lag screw (lag by technique). This was done by percutaneous

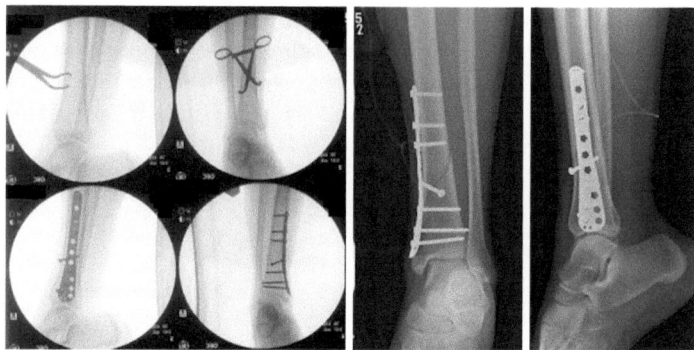

Fig. 12.2 Intraoperative and immediate postoperative imaging

means and drilled in an anterolateral to posteromedial direction.

Thereafter, the traumatic wound over the medial malleolus was extended a few centimeters proximally over the distal tibia for the placement of a neutralizing plate. The surgeon must be careful not to injure the saphenous vein or nerve during the superficial dissection. Using an elevator, a subcutaneous but extraperiosteal tunnel was developed over the medial tibia for plate insertion in a tissue-sparing fashion. The reduction clamp was removed at this time, and the plate was inserted and provisionally held with K-wires. After fluoroscopic verification of plate position, a total of six 3.5 mm screws were inserted into the plate with bicortical fixation. The three distal screws (variable-angle locking) were inserted under direct visualization, while the proximal screws (nonlocking) were placed percutaneously under fluoroscopic guidance (immediate postoperative radiographs are shown). The wound was closed over a drain positioned near the fracture site (Fig. 12.2).

Postoperative Plan

A long leg plaster splint was placed, and the patient was instructed to be non-weight-bearing on the left lower extremity. Antibiotics were continued for a total of 48 h after presentation to the trauma bay.

On serial examinations, the patient had soft compartments and stable neurologic findings. Low molecular weight heparin and a right lower extremity sequential compression device were utilized for venous thromboembolism prophylaxis. The drain was discontinued when the output was less than 30 cc per nursing shift.

A postoperative noncontrast CT scan was obtained to further evaluate the left tibial plateau fracture pattern, and later in the hospital course, the patient returned to the operating room for tibial plateau open reduction and internal fixation. She was allowed to toe-touch weight-bear 2 weeks after surgery and was progressed to weight-bearing as tolerated at 3 months.

Outcome

The patient has been followed in the office, and her 15-month postoperative radiographs are shown in Fig. 12.3. They demonstrate union of the distal tibial fracture in anatomic alignment without hardware complication. She completed a course of physical therapy and has been weight-bearing as tolerated without assistive device (Fig. 12.3).

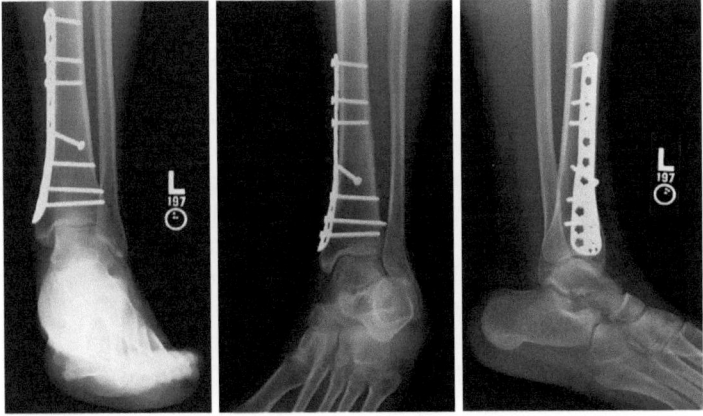

Fig. 12.3 Fifteen-month postoperative radiographs

Salient Points/Pearls

- Tibial shaft fractures are among the more common open injuries and highly associated with compartment syndrome. The surgeon must have a high index of suspicion for these conditions at the time of initial evaluation and treatment.
- Several prospective studies have been conducted comparing distal tibial shaft fixation with intramedullary nails versus open reduction and plate fixation. Both methods of fixation have good union rates, with plate fixation resulting in less angular deformity, but with possibly a higher incidence of wound complications and hardware removal [1–3].
- Open reduction and plate fixation can have several advantages over an intramedullary nail, including increased construct stiffness under axial load (especially along the near-cortex adjacent to the plate), greater ability to utilize an absolute stability construct when applicable (e.g., long oblique fracture with minimal comminution), more options for fixation of very distal fragments (especially in the setting of intraarticular fracture extension), and lack of trauma to the knee or proximal tibia (e.g., in the setting of concomitant ipsilateral tibial plateau injury). Plates may be inserted in a minimally invasive subcutaneous fashion that preserves soft tissues and vascular supply (intramedullary and periosteal) to the fracture site [1–3].
- When evaluating a patient with distal tibial shaft fracture, if there is concern for an intraarticular component, obtain dedicated ankle radiographs and consider a CT scan for further evaluation. Extension of the fracture into the articular surface of the ankle could influence the surgical plan.
- An intact fibula (or anatomically reduced fibula fracture) can greatly facilitate reduction of the tibial shaft fracture. It helps gauge appropriate tibial length, prevents varus/valgus deformity with medial-sided plating, and is necessary to stabilize the ankle in the setting of syndesmotic injury. The fibula can be fixed with a plate or intramedullary wire, depending on the fracture pattern [4].

References

1. Zelle BA, Bhandari M, Espiritu M, Koval KJ, Zlowodzki M, Evidence-Base Orthopaedic Trauma Working Group. Treatment of distal tibia fracture without articular involvement: a systematic review of 1125 fractures. J Orthop Trauma. 2006;20(1):76–9.
2. Guo JJ, Tang N, Yang HL, Tang TS. A prospective, randomized trial comparing closed intramedullary nailing with percutaneous plating in the treatment of distal metaphyseal fractures of the tibia. J Bone Joint Surg Br. 2010;92(7):984–8.
3. Vallier HA, Cureton BA, Patterson BM. Randomized, prospective comparison of plate versus intramedullary nail fixation for distal tibia shaft fractures. J Orthop Trauma. 2011;25(12):736–41.
4. Egol KA, Weisz R, Hiebert R, Tejwani NC, Koval KJ, Sander RW. Does fibular plating improve alignment after intramedullary nailing of the distal metaphyseal tibia fractures? J Orthop Trauma. 2006;20(2):94–103.

Chapter 13
Tibia Shaft Fractures of the Distal Third Treated with Plate Fixation of Tibia and Fibula

Elliott J. Kim and A. Alex Jahangir

Case Presentation

This is a 28-year-old female who sustained a closed left distal tibial shaft fracture with an associated fibular fracture following a twisting injury to her leg. Initially the patient was placed in a long leg splint in the Emergency Department to stabilize her fractured tibia and fibula, with plans to conduct operative fixation. Upon presentation, the physical exam demonstrated that the patient was neurovascularly intact and did not have any evidence of compartment syndrome.

Injury Films

AP, lateral, and oblique radiographs of the left ankle reveal an extra-articular spiral fracture of the distal third of the tibia with an associated fibular fracture (Fig. 13.1).

E.J. Kim, MD • A.A. Jahangir, MD, MMHC (✉)
Division of Orthopaedic Trauma, Department of Orthopaedic Surgery and Rehabilitation, Vanderbilt University Medical Center,
1215 21st Ave S Suite 4200, Nashville, TN 37232-8774, USA
e-mail: alex.jahangir@vanderbilt.edu

© Springer International Publishing Switzerland 2016   149
N.C. Tejwani (ed.), *Fractures of the Tibia: A Clinical Casebook*,
DOI 10.1007/978-3-319-21774-1_13

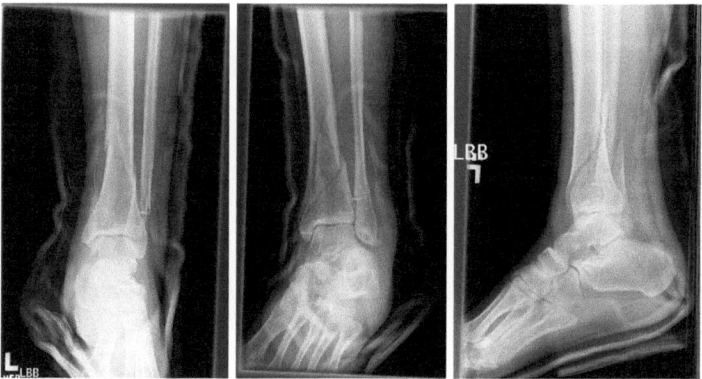

Fig. 13.1 Injury Radiographs

Treatment and Timing of Surgery

Given the fact that this is an unstable injury pattern in an active individual, the decision was made to treat the injury with open reduction and internal fixation. Due to the low energy nature of the injury, there was no significant soft tissue swelling and the surgery was performed the day after initial evaluation.

Surgical Tact

Position

Supine on a radiolucent table, with a small bump under the ipsilateral hip to allow neutral positioning of the leg. Fluoroscopy was done throughout the case with the machine coming in from the same side to allow for medial approach to the tibia.

Approach

Direct lateral over the fibula for the lateral incision.

A small incision was made over the distal medial tibia with percutaneous incisions made for the tibial shaft screws of the plate.

Fracture Reduction

The fibular reduction and fixation was conducted initially in order to facilitate reduction and alignment of the tibia through intact ligaments and soft tissue. Initial reduction of the fibular fracture was obtained using a point-to-point reduction clamp. A screw was then placed using lag technique in order to obtain and maintain compression across the fracture. A one-third tubular plate (8-hole) was placed along the lateral aspect of the fibular to serve as a neutralization plate.

After the fixation of the fibula, the reduction of the tibia was assessed. The reduction can be fine-tuned using reduction techniques including reduction clamps, Shanz pins, and possibly a femoral distractor. After the reduction of the tibia was confirmed, a small (4 cm) incision was made over the distal medial aspect of the tibia. A precontoured distal tibial plate was inserted percutaneously along the medial aspect of the tibia. The position of the plate and the reduction of the fracture were checked using fluoroscopy. Point-to-point reduction clamps can be used to aide with reduction. A cortical screw was initially placed in the most distal screw hole proximal to the fracture in order to buttress the plate to the bone, and assist in the reduction of the fracture. After this screw was placed, screws were placed in the distal tibial segment in order to secure the plate to the tibia. Once the reduction, length, alignment, and rotation of the tibia was confirmed, a total of four bicortical screws were placed in the tibial shaft using percutaneous technique, and a total of three screws were placed in the distal tibia.

Final radiographs were obtained to ensure proper reduction of the fracture before irrigating wounds and final closure (Fig. 13.2).

Postoperative Plan

The patient was initially placed in a short-leg splint with non-weight-bearing precautions. The patient's first postoperative clinic visit was 2 weeks after surgery. At this point, the patient was

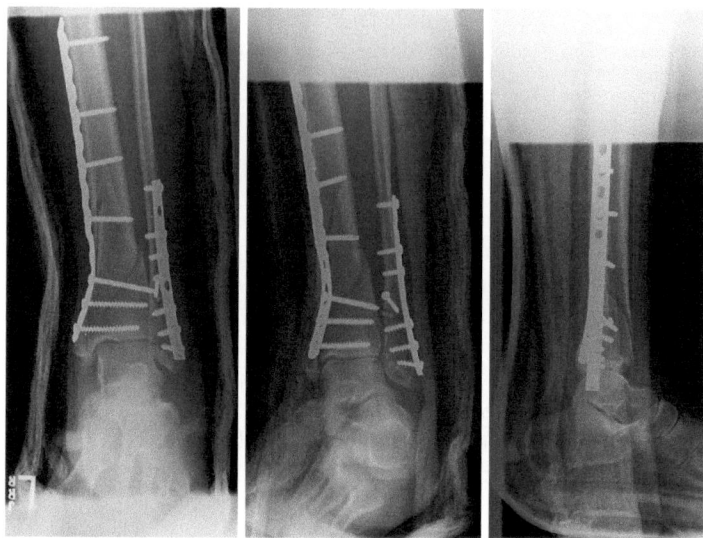

Fig. 13.2 Immediate post-operative Radiographs

transitioned into a removable splint or walking boot in order to begin ROM exercises but still remained non-weight bearing. The patient was transitioned to weight bearing as tolerated at the eight-week time frame, determined by both the clinical exam and radiographic evidence of healing.

Outcome

Approximately 6 months after her injury and surgery, radiographic imaging showed the fracture to be well healed (Fig. 13.3). The patient returned to full weight bearing without limitations and did not require any pain medications. She did, however, complain of dull "achy" pain overlying her hardware and had requested subsequent hardware removal 16 months after her initial fixation. She underwent hardware removal and did well postoperatively and was satisfied with her outcome.

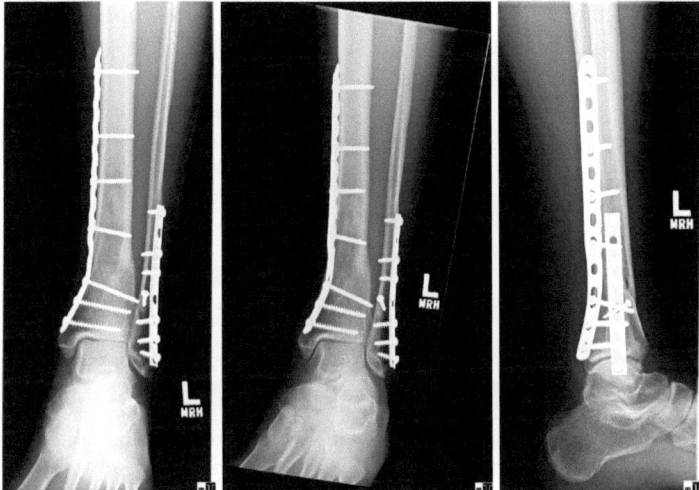

Fig. 13.3 5-month post-operative radiographs

Complications

Subsequent hardware removal 16 months postoperatively secondary to irritation from underlying hardware.

Salient Points/Pearls

- Initial fixation of the fibula fracture is useful to help with initial reduction and to regain length prior to fixation of the tibia.
- It is critical that the fibular reduction and fixation is correct, or one may have difficulty obtaining the reduction of the tibia fracture. For this reason, one may consider obtaining temporary reduction and stabilization but delaying definitive fixation of the fibula until after the tibia is reduced and stabilized.
- Point-to-point reduction clamps are a useful tool to help maintain reduction prior to plate fixation.
- Intramedullary nailing is another option for operative fixation of extra-articular distal tibia fractures that provides comparable outcomes.

- Intramedullary nailing may prove to be a better option if there is significant soft tissue injury and concern for wound complications with incisions in the zone of injury.
- Complications to consider with these specific injuries outside of nonunion, malunion, and hardware infection include prominent hardware and associated pain which lead to reoperation for hardware removal.

References

1. Kwok CS, Crossman PT, Loizou CL. Plate versus nail for distal tibial fractures: a systematic review and meta-analysis. J Orthop Trauma. 2014;28:542–8.
2. Li B, Yang Y, Jiang LS. Plate fixation versus intramedullary nailing for displaced extra-articular distal tibia fractures: a system review. Eur J Orthop Surg Traumatol. 2015;25:53–63.
3. Sathiyakumar V, Thakore RV, Ihejirika RC, Obremskey WT, Sethi MK. Distal tibia fractures and medial plating: factors influencing re-operation. Int Orthop. 2014;38:1483–8.
4. Berlusconi M, Busnelli L, Chiodini F, Portinaro N. To fix or not to fix? The role of fibular fixation in distal shaft fractures of the leg. Injury. 2014;45(2):408–11.

Part III
Treatment of Open Tibia Fractures

Chapter 14
Open Tibia Fractures: Staged Treatment

William Min

Clinical History/Scenario

This is a 24-year-old male without significant past medical or surgical history who was involved in an isolated motorcycle accident. He presented to the trauma bay with a right open proximal third tibial shaft fracture. There were no other reported injuries. He reports only pain about the affected extremity that is relieved with administered analgesics.

On physical examination, the patient is afebrile and vital signs are within normal limits. Secondary examination does not reveal any further abnormalities. Evaluation of the affected extremity reveals a 5-cm laceration centered anteriorly over the fracture site. The fracture is clearly visible through the open wound. There is mild contamination. His compartments are soft on palpation. Range of motion was not tested given his injuries, but he is able to demonstrate ability to move his ankle and toes grossly. There is no evidence of sensory or motor deficit on neurological examination of the leg. He has lack of palpable/dopplerable pulse along the dorsalis

W. Min, MD, MS, MBA
The Hughston Clinic at Gwinnett Medical Center, Lawrenceville, GA, USA
e-mail: min.william@gmail.com

© Springer International Publishing Switzerland 2016 157
N.C. Tejwani (ed.), *Fractures of the Tibia: A Clinical Casebook*,
DOI 10.1007/978-3-319-21774-1_14

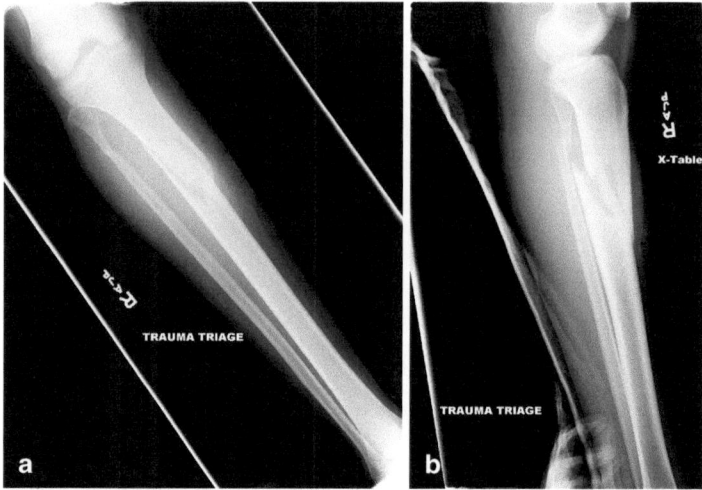

Fig. 14.1 AP (**a**) and lateral (**b**) radiographs of proximal third tibial shaft fracture

and posterior tibia arteries; these are not symmetric to the contralateral side.

Imaging evaluation reveals that he has a proximal third tibial shaft fracture (Fig. 14.1a, b).

Treatment Considerations/Planning/Tests Needed

This patient presents with an isolated injury to the right tibia. The concerning findings currently are that he has an open tibial fracture with asymmetric pulses. The first treatment consideration here is to initiate empiric antibiotic therapy (to lessen the risk of infection) and to perform closed reduction, as his displacement may account for his pulse discrepancy.

Unfortunately, after reduction was achieved, the pulse exam did not improve. A CT angiogram was performed, which revealed loss of flow proximal to the bifurcation of the popliteal artery. At this point, vascular consultation is required, as vascular repair may be necessary. Discussion with the vascular team is necessary, as this will guide the decision to either treat this injury definitively or with temporization measures (external fixation) during the initial irrigation and debridement.

The CT scan is also beneficial here, as it helps identify the presence of a proximal intra-articular extension of the fracture (which may alter treatment management decisions). The presence of intra-articular extension may warrant additional compression screw fixation in the setting of intramedullary nail (IMN) fixation or, alternatively, open reduction with plate(s) and screws should IMN fixation not be possible.

Additionally, discussions should be held with the trauma team regarding physiologic status. While this is a single-limb injury, the presence of vascular injury implies a high-energy mechanism. This, coupled with the potential need for resuscitation, may prohibit early definitive treatment to prevent the "second hit" to the patient's system.

Timing of Surgery

Given the open nature of this injury, it requires urgent treatment with irrigation and debridement, coupled with surgical stabilization (either in the form of definitive fixation versus temporization). The vascular team concluded, based on the findings of the CT angiogram, that he requires vascular repair. For this reason, he cannot proceed with definitive fixation, and would be best served with external fixation for temporization. Controversy exists as to when external fixation should proceed in the timing of vascular repair, as there is literature to support both modalities (before and after vascular repair). This decision should be based on the warm versus cold ischemia time, the severity of the displacement (as significant reduction maneuvers may potentially disrupt the vascular repair), and the extent/manner of the vascular repair (which could be hindered by the external fixator placement).

After discussions with the vascular team, because the limb was still warm and there were concerns regarding the potential for vascular repair disruption with reductive manipulation, we

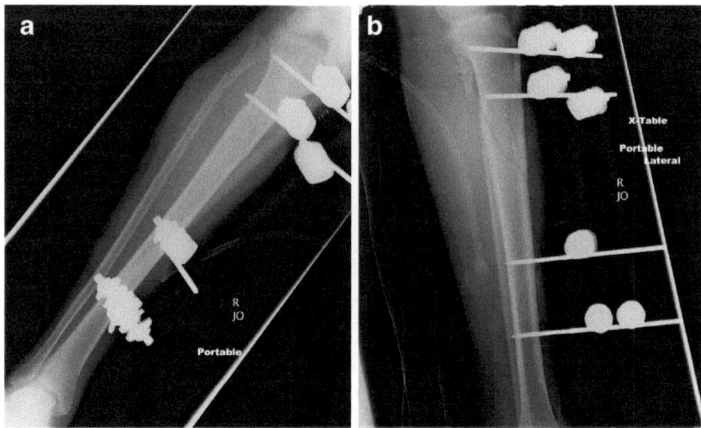

Fig. 14.2 AP (**a**) and lateral (**b**) radiographs of proximal third tibial shaft fracture, status post I&D and external fixation

proceeded first with irrigation and debridement of his open fracture with fracture stabilization via external fixation (Fig. 14.2a, b). A prophylactic dual-incision fasciotomy was performed after the vascular repair. There was no significant skin loss, thus permitting primary repair of the traumatic laceration. He was placed on long-term antibiotic coverage, as he had an open medial fasciotomy site; otherwise, coverage would be limited to 48 h of antibiotic coverage.

Intraoperative Tips and Tricks for Reduction/ Fixation

Because of the presence of vascular repair in the setting of an open fracture, this injury is classified as a Gustilo-Anderson type IIIC open injury. The considerations for the definitive construct should be based on the fracture pattern and the nature of his vascular repair. Proximal third tibial shaft fractures can be sufficiently addressed with IMN fixation, with attention paid toward the appropriate lateral start point (to avoid valgus and procurvatum deformities typically seen with malpositioned start points). The addition of blocking and/or positioning screws can also aid both fracture reduction and construct stability [1, 2].

However, in discussions with the vascular team, their repair warrants that the patient be limited from knee range of motion for 3–6 weeks. While this does preclude infrapatellar IMN insertion, suprapatellar or semiextended IMN insertion is still permissible. In his case, we elected to perform open reduction internal fixation with plate and screws (Fig. 14.3a–d) as opposed to semiextended IMN insertion, given the presence of an open fracture site (which permitted us to obtain anatomic restoration for an absolute stability construct) and the inability to perform knee range of motion. We obtained anatomic restoration of his fracture site with stabilization via lag screw compression and neutralization plate fixation. While IMN is a favorable tactic in the setting of open fasciotomy wounds (to lessen the risk of implant contamination), we were able to primarily close the fasciotomy wounds (medially with primary closure, laterally with split thickness skin grafting) at the time of definitive fixation.

Postoperative Protocols

IMN fixation may permit earlier weight bearing as opposed to plate and screw constructs, and, for this reason, we withheld his weight bearing for 12 weeks. He was allowed to initiate knee range of motion after this was cleared by vascular surgery (at the 3-week mark). He was placed on 48 h of antibiotic prophylaxis after definitive fixation. He was placed on DVT prophylaxis until he was able to adequately mobilize and ambulate to the contralateral extremity.

Follow-Up

He was evaluated by us at the 3-week, 12-week (Fig. 14.4a, b), 6-month, and 1-year time points (Fig. 14.5a, b). At his 1-year follow-up, he was ambulating independently and asymptomatically without any gait, function, or range of motion limitations.

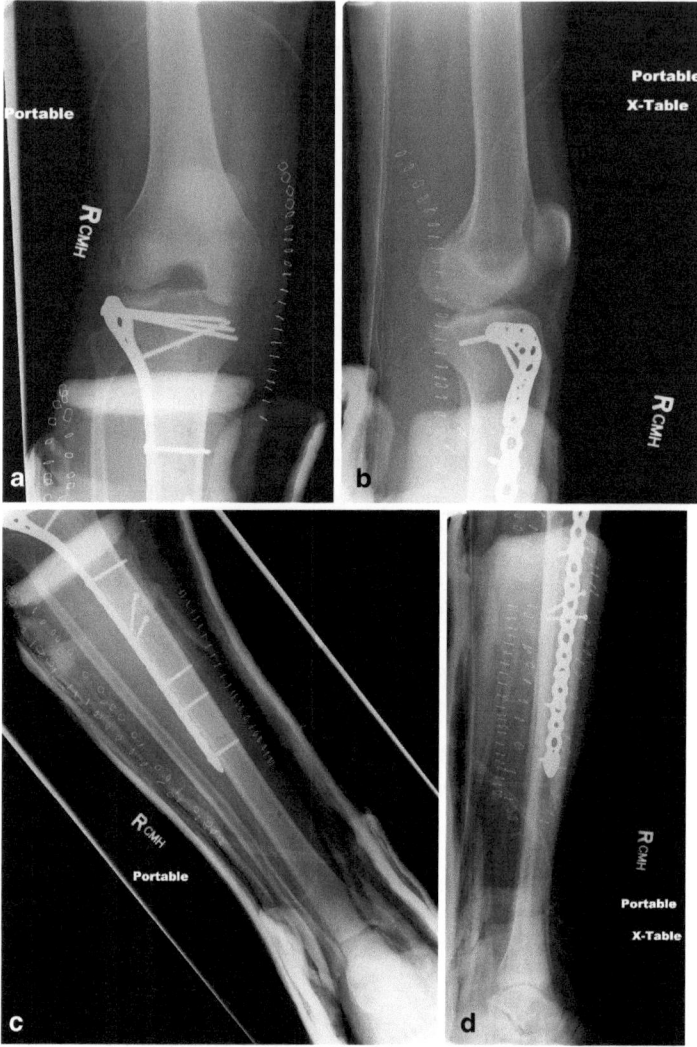

Fig. 14.3 AP (**a**, **c**) and lateral (**b**, **d**) radiographs of proximal third tibial shaft fracture, status post ORIF

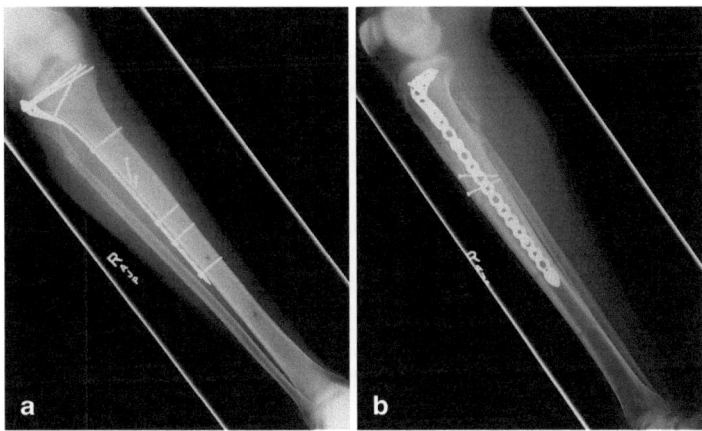

Fig. 14.4 AP (**a**) and lateral (**b**) radiographs of proximal third tibial shaft fracture, 12 weeks status post definitive fixation

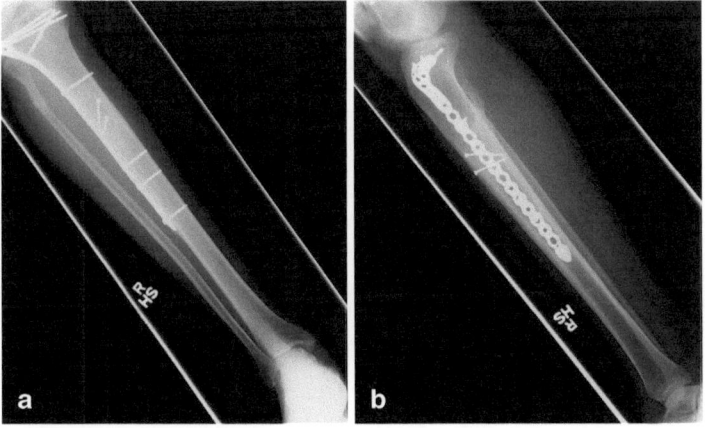

Fig. 14.5 AP (**a**) and lateral (**b**) radiographs of proximal third tibial shaft fracture, 1 year status post definitive fixation

Salient Points/Pearls

- Open proximal third tibia fractures are caused by high-energy mechanisms and associated with vascular or neurological injuries and compartment syndrome.
- Use of an external fixator is warranted in setting where vascular repair is needed; the usual protocol is limb revascularization followed by bony stabilization; though this may be modified on a case-by-case basis as was done here.
- Definitive fixation can be achieved once the vascular repair is stable; timing for definitive fixation should be made in conjunction with discussions with the vascular team.

References

1. Krettek C, Miclau T, Schandelmaier P, Stephan C, Möhlmann U, Tscherne H. The mechanical effect of blocking screws ('Poller screws') in stabilizing tibia fractures with short proximal or distal fragments after insertion of small-diameter intramedullary nails. J Orthop Trauma. 1999;13(8):550–3.
2. Ricci WM, O'Boyle M, Borrelli J, Bellabarba C, Sanders R. Fractures of the proximal third of the tibial shaft treated with intramedullary nails and blocking screws. J Orthop Trauma. 2001;15(4):264–70.

Chapter 15
Open Tibial Fracture with Immediate Fixation and Early Soft Tissue Coverage

Daniel N. Segina

Case Presentation

This is a 35-year-old male involved in a motorcycle collision. The patient was brought in as a trauma alert where he was noted to have injuries isolated to his right lower extremity, including an open distal tibia fracture, distal fibular fracture, and medial malleolar fracture. Exposed bone and soft tissue, including tendonous structures, were noted. His wounds were dressed sterilely and he was given appropriate prophylactic IV antibiotics. A short leg splint was applied.

D.N. Segina, MD
Director of Orthopaedic Trauma, Holmes Regional Trauma Center, Melbourne, FL, USA

Assistant Professor, University of Central Florida College of Medicine, Orlando, FL, USA
e-mail: dsegina@cfl.rr.com

© Springer International Publishing Switzerland 2016   165
N.C. Tejwani (ed.), *Fractures of the Tibia: A Clinical Casebook*,
DOI 10.1007/978-3-319-21774-1_15

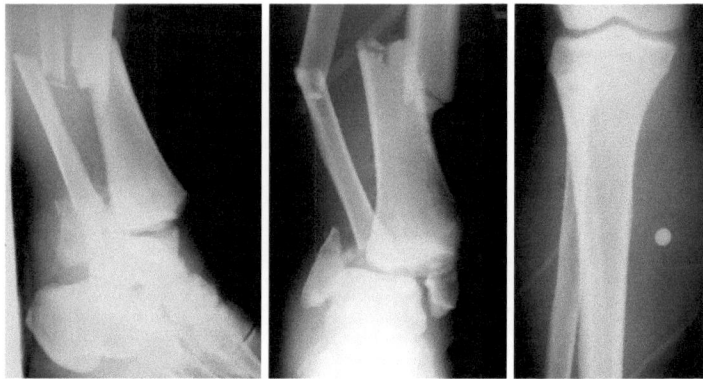

Fig. 15.1 Injury radiographs

Injury Films

AP and lateral (Fig. 15.1) demonstrated a comminuted fracture of
the distal tibia and fibula with noncontiguous segmental fibula and
medial malleolar involvement consistent with a local crush injury.

Treatment and Timing of Surgery

The treatment plan was based upon multiple factors, the most important of which was the degree of contamination and the underlying
fracture pattern. Surgical debridement, intramedullary stabilization of
the tibia as well as fixation of the fibula and medial malleolus was
accomplished within 6 h of presentation to the trauma center.

Surgical Plan

Position

The patient was placed supine on a radiolucent table with a towel
bump underneath the ipsilateral buttock/hip. A long offset leg

wedge was used to provide for unobstructed access to the distal tibia, fibula, medial malleolus, as well as soft tissue injury. Additionally, a radiolucent triangle was utilized to assist in obtaining a starting portal and nail insertion.

Surgical Approach

The open fracture was first addressed utilizing a formal surgical debridement. Traumatic wounds were surgically extended in a manner to allow for appropriate exposure of the underlying bone and soft tissue, while not compromising future soft tissue coverage. Nonviable tissue was surgically excised. Priority was given to retaining neurovascular structures, tendonous structures, as well as bone with soft tissue attachment. The exposed tissue and bone were cleansed using multiple liters of sterile saline at low pressure. Once the debridement was completed, attention was shifted to obtaining an appropriate starting portal for the nail insertion. A patellar tendon splitting approach was chosen. The segmental fibular injury was addressed through a lateral exposure separate from the traumatic wound. The medial malleolar injury was addressed through the traumatic open wound allowing for direct reduction and screw fixation.

Fracture Reduction/Implant Insertion

The reduction was assisted by anatomical reduction of the segmental fibular fracture prior to nail insertion. The medial malleolar component of the injury was not addressed at this time. Once the fibular anatomy had been restored, further reduction of the tibial component of the injury was accomplished with manual manipulation and clamp application. A guide wire was advanced into the distal metaphysis, where sequential reaming to 1.5 mm over the chosen nail diameter was performed. The chosen nail diameter was determined at the time of surgery based upon resistance to reamer passing through the tibial isthmus and the presence of bone debris on the reamer head. The smallest diameter nail to accomplish this was chosen. This allows for the least amount of medullary blood flow disturbance, heat generation from reaming, and provides an opportunity for exchange nailing should a delayed union or nonunion arise. Interlocking screws were inserted with attention focused on the prevention of any excessive distraction at the tibial fracture site. Two distal interlocking screws were used based upon the infraisthmal location of the tibial shaft fracture. One static interlock was used proximally. Finally, the medial malleolus was repaired with the use of retrograde cannulated lag screws (Fig. 15.2).

Wound Management

Surgical incisions were closed primarily after thorough inspection for hemostasis and final irrigation. The traumatic open wounds were managed with the use of a negative pressure wound dressing (Fig. 15.3). Repeat surgical debridements of the open wounds were performed at 72 h intervals. The negative pressure wound dressing was replaced at that time. Definitive soft tissue coverage was accomplished at postinjury day 9, noting a clean wound with healthy granulation tissue (Fig. 15.4). A reverse flow sural artery fasciocutaneous flap was chosen as well as split thickness skin graft (Fig. 15.5). Antibiotics were continued until definitive soft tissue coverage was achieved.

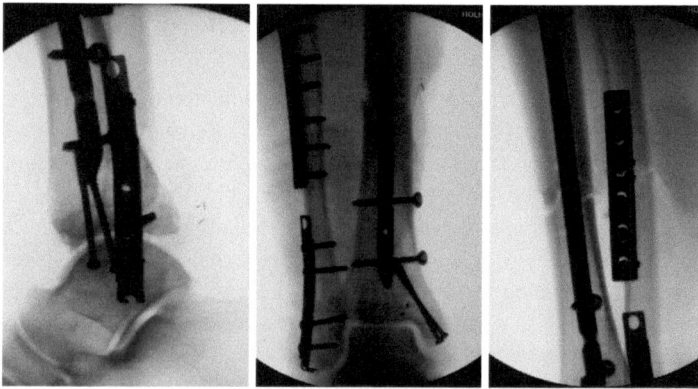

Fig. 15.2 Intraoperative radiographs after immediate fixation

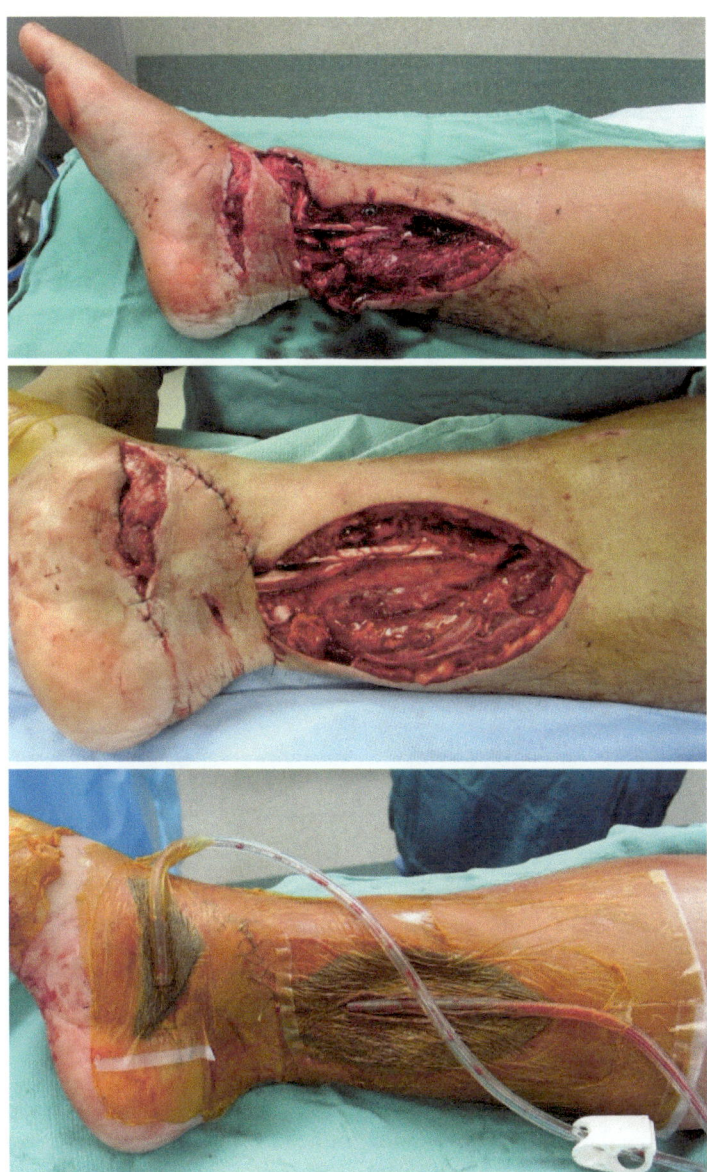

Fig. 15.3 Initial wound and NPWT management

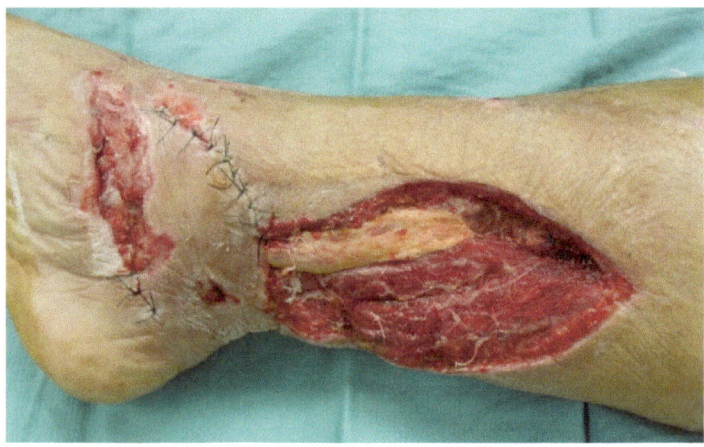

Fig. 15.4 POD # 9 wound appearance

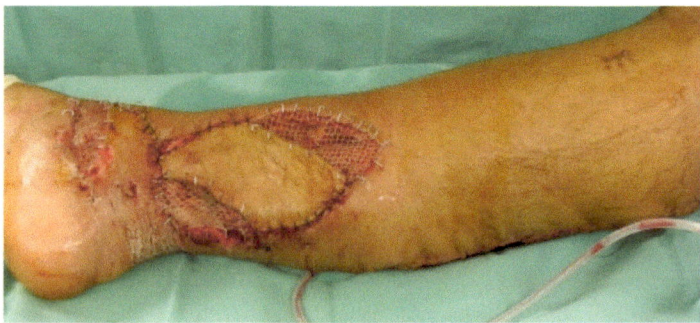

Fig. 15.5 POD # 9 medial wound after sural artery pedicle flap and STSG

Postoperative Plan

Full range of motion of the knee was allowed beginning postoperative day 1. Range of motion of the ankle was restricted for two weeks to allow for sural flap healing. Dressing changes were performed until staples and sutures were removed at two weeks post sural flap coverage, at which time full range of motion of the foot and ankle was allowed. Because of the ipsilateral fibular and medial malleolar fractures, a postoperative non-weight-bearing restriction was imposed. Progressive weight bearing was begun 6 weeks postoperatively.

Outcome

The patient was seen monthly, with follow-up radiographs. Radiographs performed at the 8-month postoperative visit revealed no progression of healing, consistent with nonunion of the tibial shaft component of the injury. The fibula, as well as medial malleolus, was noted to be healed (Fig. 15.6) There were no clinical signs of infection; however, serologic studies were ordered to assess the potential for underlying infection. White blood cell count, erythrocyte sedimentation rate, as well as C-reactive protein were all noted to be normal. An exchange tibial nailing was performed enlarging the nail size by 2 mm. The nail was interlocked using two distal screws. No proximal interlocking screws were utilized to provide for dynamic fixation. Prominent, painful hardware at the fibula and medial malleolus was removed at that time. Follow-up radiographs 2.5 years post injury demonstrated bony union (Fig. 15.7). Prominent hardware at the proximal tibia nail insertion site as well as the distal interlocking screw site prompted removal of the remaining implants (Fig. 15.8). The patient obtained excellent cosmesis (Fig. 15.9) and functional recovery including the ability to participate in CrossFit training as well as running and cycling.

Complications

Nonunion surgically treated at 8 months, and hardware irritation requiring surgical removal.

Teaching Points

Open fractures of the lower extremity mandate a well thought out plan for skeletal stabilization as well as soft tissue management.

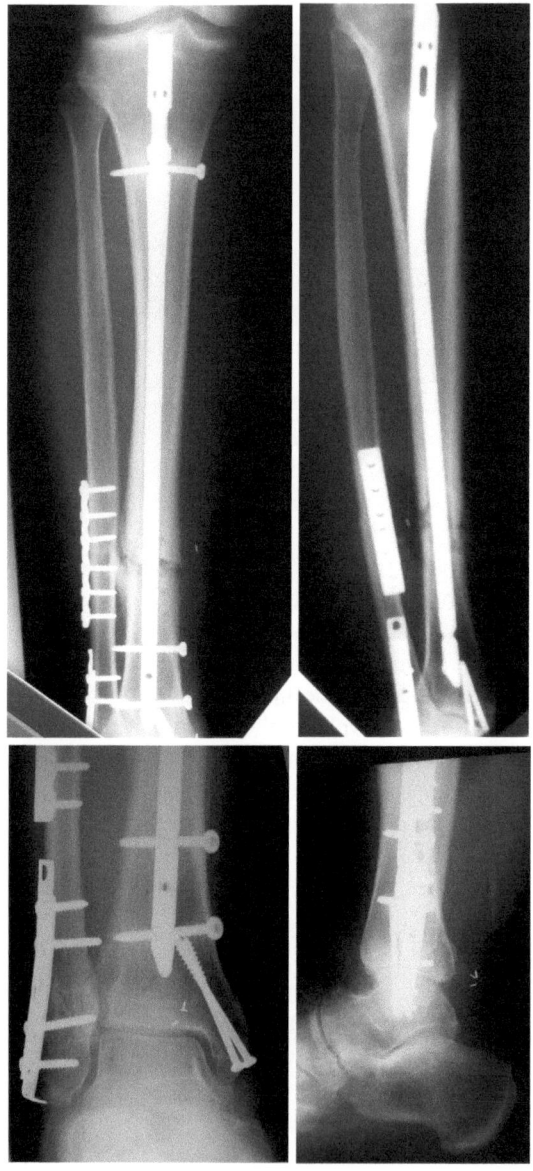

Fig. 15.6 Eight-month postoperative radiographs

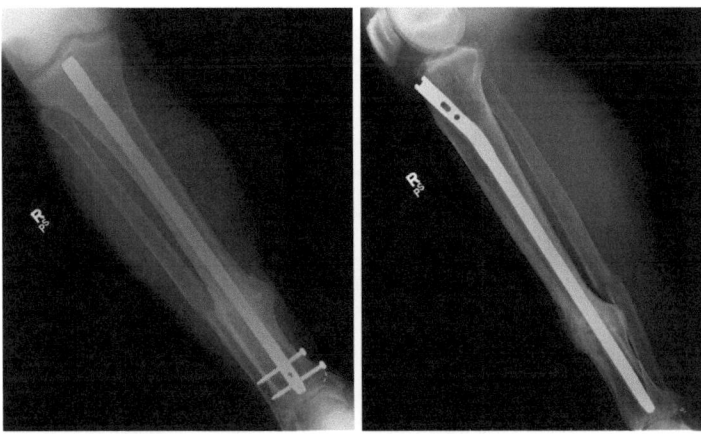

Fig. 15.7 Fracture union 1 year after exchange nailing

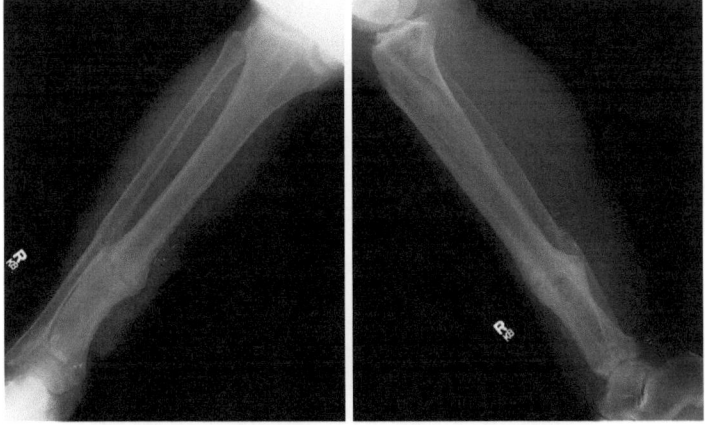

Fig. 15.8 Final radiographs after hardware removal, 2.5 years after injury

The prompt administration of IV prophylactic antibiotics is mandatory. Clean wound dressings and splint stabilization are adequate prior to the patient presenting to the operating room.

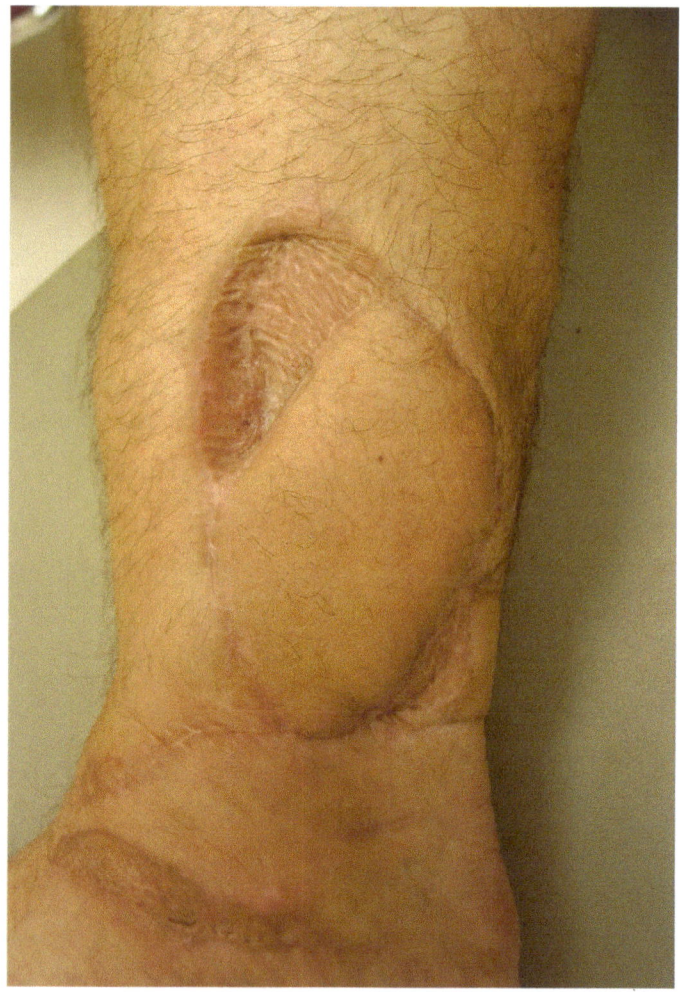

Fig. 15.9 Final clinical photo 2.5 years after injury

Once in the operating room, attention to detail is crucial, beginning with patient positioning. This facilitates surgical exposure as well as fluoroscopic visualization.

Open fracture and wound debridement should be accomplished before operative stabilization is performed. If no gross contamination is appreciated, intramedullary stabilization can be safely accomplished. Contaminated instruments should be removed from the operative field prior to nail insertion.

Anatomic restoration and stabilization of the fibula aid in reduction of the tibia. Additionally, direct visualization of the fracture site assists with tibial reduction and may be enhanced using clamp application. If an ipsilateral medial malleolar injury is present, fixation of this component of the injury is accomplished after intramedullary nail placement and interlocking screw insertion. This avoids any potential obstruction of the nail insertion into the distal tibia.

A minimum of two screws should be used for distal interlocking due to the infra-isthmal location of the fracture. A single static interlocking screw should be placed proximally for rotational control and to prevent any excessive shortening.

Negative pressure wound therapy can be helpful in the early management of open extremity wounds.

The postoperative rehabilitation protocol focuses initially on knee and ankle range of motion to prevent contracture. Full weight bearing can be allowed immediately postoperatively in isolated tibial fractures stabilized with a locked intramedullary nail. Injuries with concomitant complicated wounds and / or additional fractures around the ankle require a non-weight-bearing protocol to prevent early loss of fixation and excessive wound edema .

Complications are divided into acute and delayed. Acute postinjury/surgical complications include infection and loss of alignment. Delayed complications include nonunion, late infection, hardware irritation, and anterior knee pain.

Further Reading

Brinker MR, O'Connor DP. Exchange nailing of ununited fractures. J Bone Joint Surg Am. 2007;89(1):177–88.

Akhtar S, Hameed A. Versatility of the sural fasciocutaneous flap in the coverage of lower third leg and hind foot defects. J Plast Reconstr Aesthet Surg. 2006;59(8):839–45. Epub 2006 Mar 9.

Patzakis MJ, Wilkins J. Factors influencing infection rate in open fracture wounds. Clin Orthop Relat Res. 1989;243:36–40.

Stannard JP, Singanamala N, Volgas DA. Fix and flap in the era of vacuum suction devices: what do we know in terms of evidence based medicine? Injury. 2010;41(8):780–6. doi:10.1016/j.injury.2009.08.011. Epub 2010 May 14.

Papakostidis C, Kanakaris NK, Pretel J, Faour O, Morell DJ, Giannoudis PV. Prevalence of complications of open tibial shaft fractures stratified as per the Gustilo-Anderson classification. Injury. 2011;42(12):1408–15. doi:10.1016/j.injury.2011.10.015. Epub 2011 Oct 22.

Part IV
Treatment of Distal Tibia Articular Fractures

Chapter 16
Distal Tibia Pilon: Staged Fixation with an Anterolateral Plate

Charlie Jowett, Huw Edwards, and Pramod Achan

Case Presentation

This is a 23-year-old male who sustained a closed pilon fracture and an L2 burst fracture after a high-speed motorcycle accident. He underwent initial evaluation in the emergency room and was placed into an above-knee splint and treated with spinal precautions. No other injuries were noted on secondary examination and his neurological examination revealed no deficit.

Injury Films

Injury films (AP and lateral): show a comminuted plafond fracture subluxation of the right ankle. This injury is suggestive of a direct axial force (Fig. 16.1a, b).

C. Jowett, FRCS(Orth) (✉) • H. Edwards • P. Achan
Trauma and Orthopaedics, The Royal London Hospital, Bart's Health NHS Trust, Whitechapel, London E1 1BB, UK
e-mail: charliejowett@hotmail.com

© Springer International Publishing Switzerland 2016
N.C. Tejwani (ed.), *Fractures of the Tibia: A Clinical Casebook*,
DOI 10.1007/978-3-319-21774-1_16

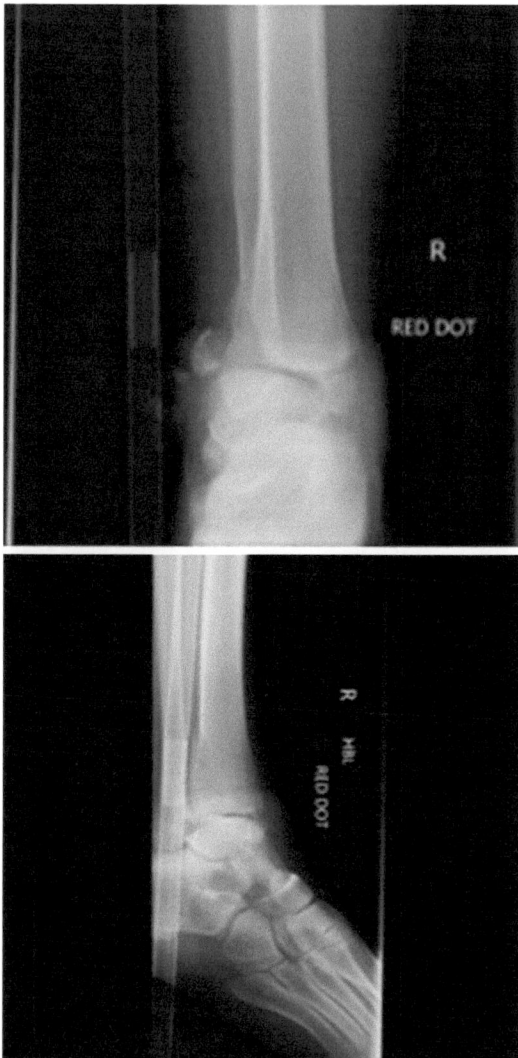

Fig. 16.1 AP and Lateral X-rays of right ankle following injury

Treatment and Timing of Surgery

CT scan in a backslab showed the joint was still subluxed. Clinically the ankle was significantly swollen. The day after admission an external fixator was applied to provide temporary stability and reduction of the tibio-talar joint [1]. Also, the length, alignment, and rotation were regained to allow for swelling to decrease. Ten days after the application of the external fixator when the soft tissues had settled this was removed and definitive open reduction and internal fixation was performed (Fig. 16.2a, b) [2].

Surgical Tact

External Fixation

Tibia on affected side placed on pillow to allow lateral X-rays without moving the leg.

"A" frame applied with a Hoffman external fixator. Two 5 mm pins were inserted in the tibia, and a 5 mm threaded Denham pin was used for the calcaneus. Another 4 mm pin was inserted at the base of the first metatarsal. A U bar was applied to frame in order to prevent heel pressure sores.

Care is taken in positioning the tibial pins proximal to the zone of injury and away from the future fixation (Fig. 16.3a, b).

Definitive Open Reduction and Internal Fixation

Once the definitive fixation was planned, the external fixator was initially removed. The medial malleolus fragment was fixed first. The fragment was held reduced with pointed reduction forceps, two 40 mm partially threaded cancellous screws secured the fragment.

The comminuted pilon fracture fixation was achieved using an anterolateral approach [3]. The superficial peroneal nerve was identified. The articular surface was restored(?) to a reduced

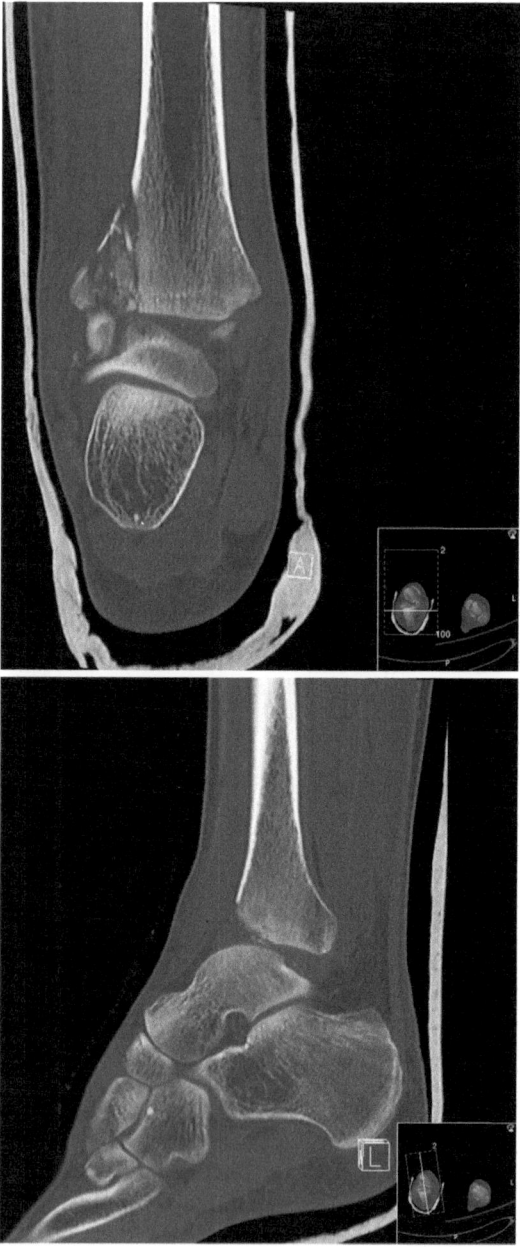

Fig. 16.2 CT scan of right ankle showing a subluxed comminuted tibial plafond fracture

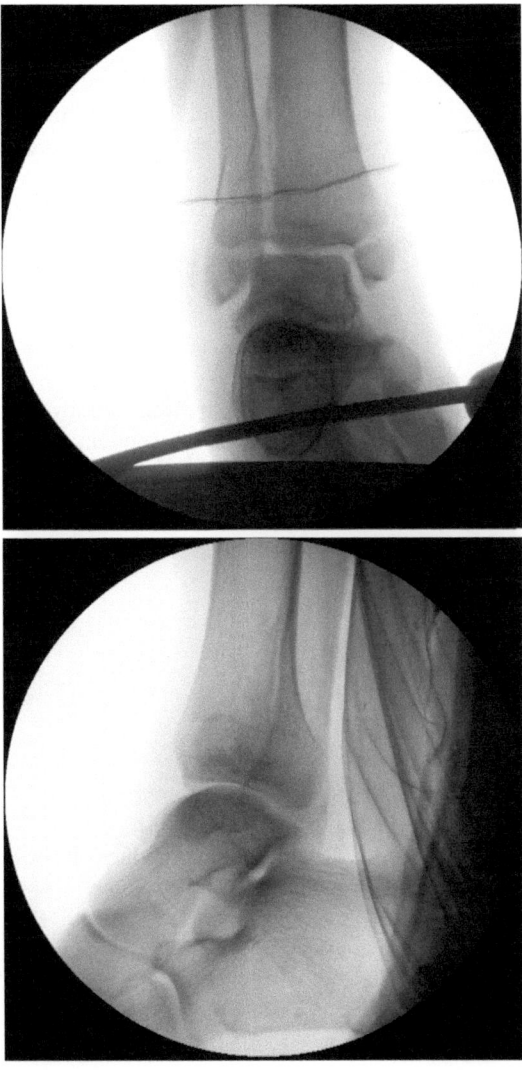

Fig. 16.3 Intraoperative X-rays of right ankle in external fixator showing the ankle joint reduced

position under fluoroscopy and held with two partially threaded cancellous screws.

Once the joint was secured an anterolateral distal tibia locking was plate applied. This was fixed with four proximal screws (two cortical screws applied before two locking screws) and three distal locking screws.

Final radiographs show fracture reduced with plate and screws in place (Fig. 16.4a, b).

Postoperative Plan

A below-knee posterior splint was applied initially and this was changed to a full plaster after 3 days. The patient was maintained non weight bearing for a period of 6 weeks in plaster. Clinical and radiographic follow-up was done until union.

Complications

None

Radiographs
1. Injury fims: AP/lateral
2. CT scan to help plan surgery is advisable
3. Intraoperative fluoroscopy to confirm reduction for both external fixation and definitive fixation
4. Post operative films
5. Follow up films at union

Salient Points/Pearls

• Prior to definitive fixation it is advisable that the soft tissues are allowed to rest by applying an external fixator. A "U" bar should be applied. This will prevent pressure sores on the heel.

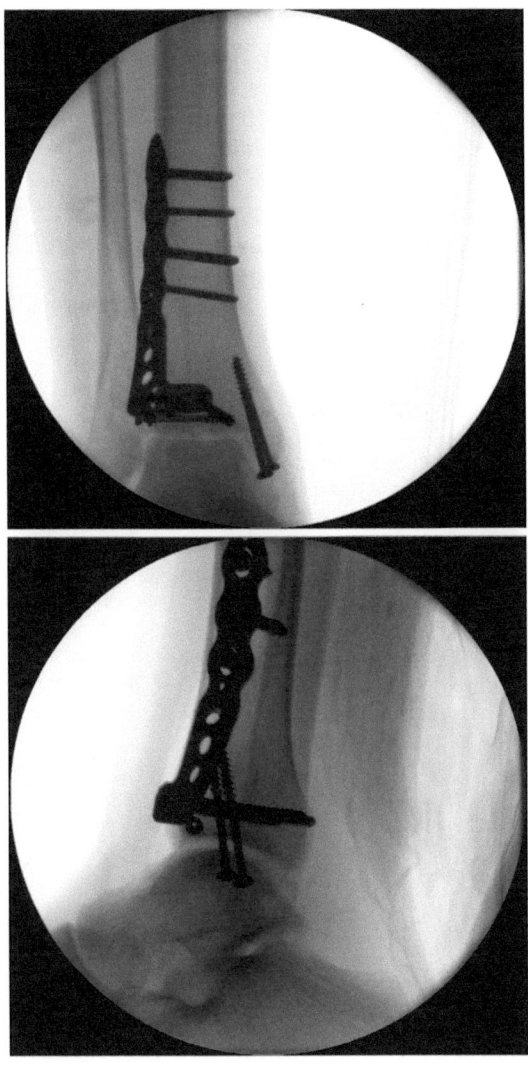

Fig. 16.4 Intraoperative X-rays showing definitive fracture fixation

- If there is significant comminution, individual fragments can be held and reduced with lag screws/K wires prior to applying the plate.
- The external fixator can be left on when performing the definitive surgery. This may help with the reduction of the fracture.
- Definitive fixation with a fine wire external fixator can also be contemplated with these fractures.
- Complications include prominent metalwork and the need for removal, infection, and nonunion.
- If the articular surface is not reduced osteoarthritis is likely to develop causing pain and ankle stiffness.

References

1. Tang X, Liu L, Tu CQ, Li J, Li Q, Pei FX. Comparison of early and delayed open reduction and internal fixation for treating closed tibial pilon fractures. Foot Ankle Int. 2014;35(7):657–64.
2. Liporace FA, Mehta S, Rhorer AS, Yoon RS, Reilly MC. Staged treatment and associated complications of pilon fractures. Instr Course Lect. 2012;61:53–70.
3. Assal M, Ray A, Stern R. Strategies for surgical approaches in open reduction internal fixation of pilon fractures. J Orthop Trauma. 2015;29(2): 69–79.

Chapter 17
Distal Tibial Pilon Fracture: Delayed Treatment and Dual Incision Approach

Richard S. Yoon, David K. Galos, and Frank A. Liporace

Case Presentation

This is a 38-year-old male, who sustained a closed injury to his left distal tibia after a fall from a 22 foot scaffold while at work. He was brought to the emergency room for evaluation and underwent placement into a long leg splint.

Initial Injury Films

Initial injury films (Fig. 17.1a, b) exhibit an intra-articular distal tibia fracture with concomitant fibula fracture and metadiaphyseal tibia comminution.

R.S. Yoon, MD (✉) • D.K. Galos, MD • F.A. Liporace, MD
Division of Orthopaedic Trauma, Department of Orthopaedic Surgery,
NYU Hospital for Joint Diseases, New York, NY, USA
e-mail: yoonrich@gmail.com

© Springer International Publishing Switzerland 2016
N.C. Tejwani (ed.), *Fractures of the Tibia: A Clinical Casebook*,
DOI 10.1007/978-3-319-21774-1_17

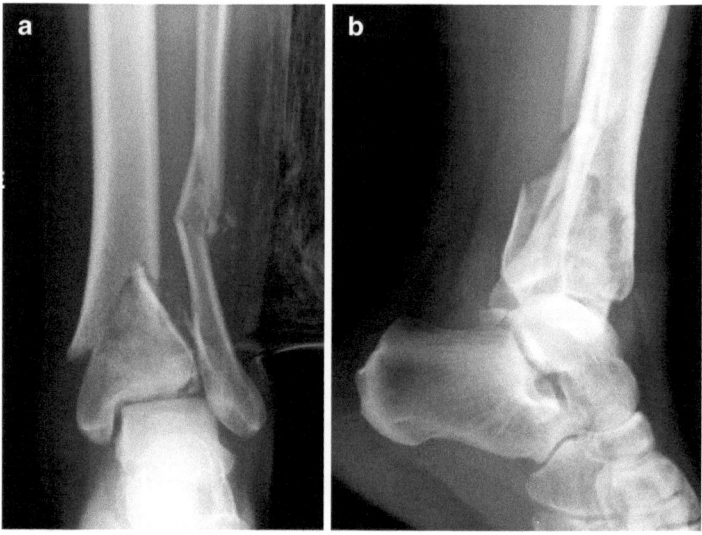

Fig. 17.1 (**a–b**) AP and lateral radiographs depicting intra-articular distal tibia fracture with concomitant fibula fracture

Treatment and Timing of Temporizing Surgery

Due to significant soft tissue swelling, the high-energy mechanism of injury, and significant comminution, the patient was placed in an external fixator a few hours after presentation (Fig. 17.2a, b).

Postexternal Fixation CT Scan

Postexternal fixation CT scan (Fig. 17.3a–i) shows severe comminution of the articular surface. Axial images (Fig. 17.3a, b) also show entrapped flexor tendons posteromedially (Fig. 17.3b). On the coronal reconstructions (Fig. 17.3c–f), moving from posterior (Fig. 17.3c) to anterior (Fig. 17.3f), severe bone loss in the metaphysis is noted along with cortical bone loss medially (Fig. 17.3e). The degrees of articular fragmentation and metaphyseal bone loss can further be appreciated on the sagittal reconstructions (Fig. 17.3g–i).

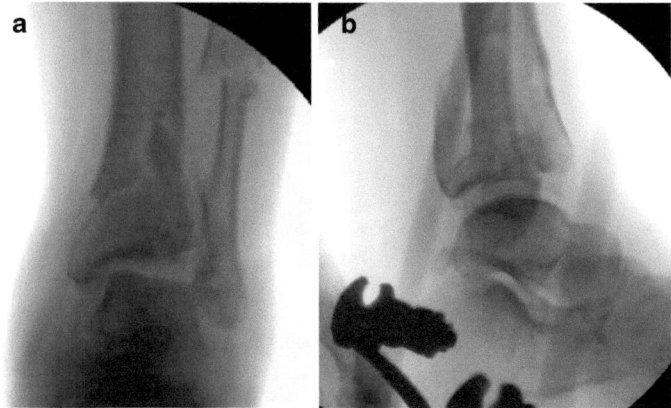

Fig. 17.2 (**a–b**) Fluoroscopic images post-external fixator placement with improved alignment, length and rotation

Treatment and Timing of Definitive Surgery

Once soft tissue swelling subsided, the decision to treat this fracture in a staged, delayed fashion was made. Approximately 1 week after injury and external fixation, the posterior half of the injury would initially be addressed and the soft tissues would be allowed to recover for another week. Finally, definitive fixation of the anterior portion of the fracture would follow in order to complete the reconstruction. The external fixator remained in place following posterior fixation as additional support to help maintain length, rotation, and alignment.

Surgical Tact

Position

For posterior fixation, the patient was placed prone. For anterior fixation, the patient was supine with bump under the ipsilateral ischial tuberosity. In both cases, the tourniquet was placed.

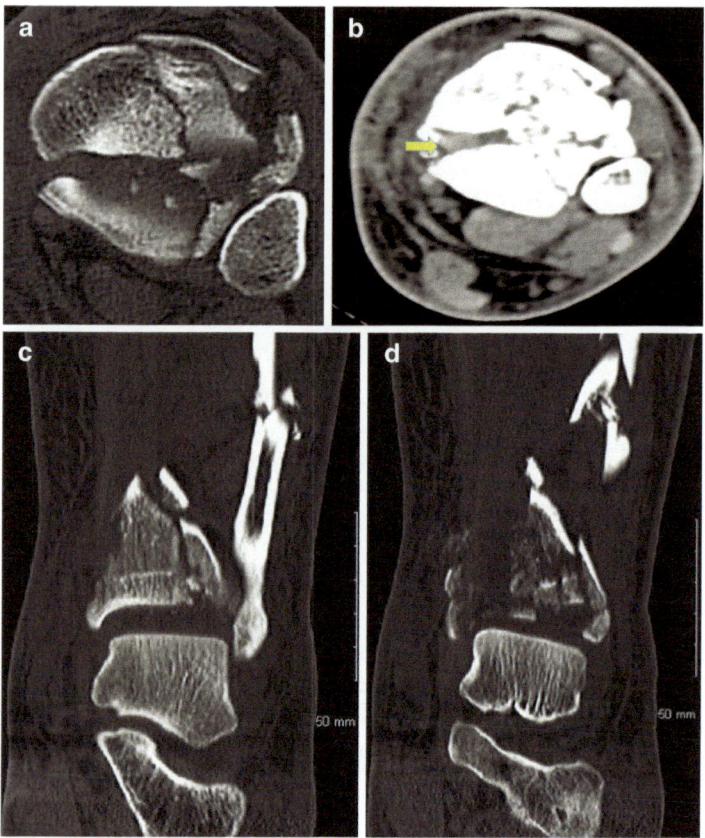

Fig. 17.3 (**a–i**) CT obtained following external fixation; comminution can be appreciated in the axial, sagittal, and coronal planes. Of note, entrapped soft tissue structures can be appreciated posteromedially (**b**)

Approach

For posterior fixation, a posterolateral approach was used to address both the fibula and the posterior half of the distal tibia. An additional, mini incision was placed posteromedially to remove the entrapped soft tissue structures from the fracture site. For anterior fixation, an anterolateral approach was used.

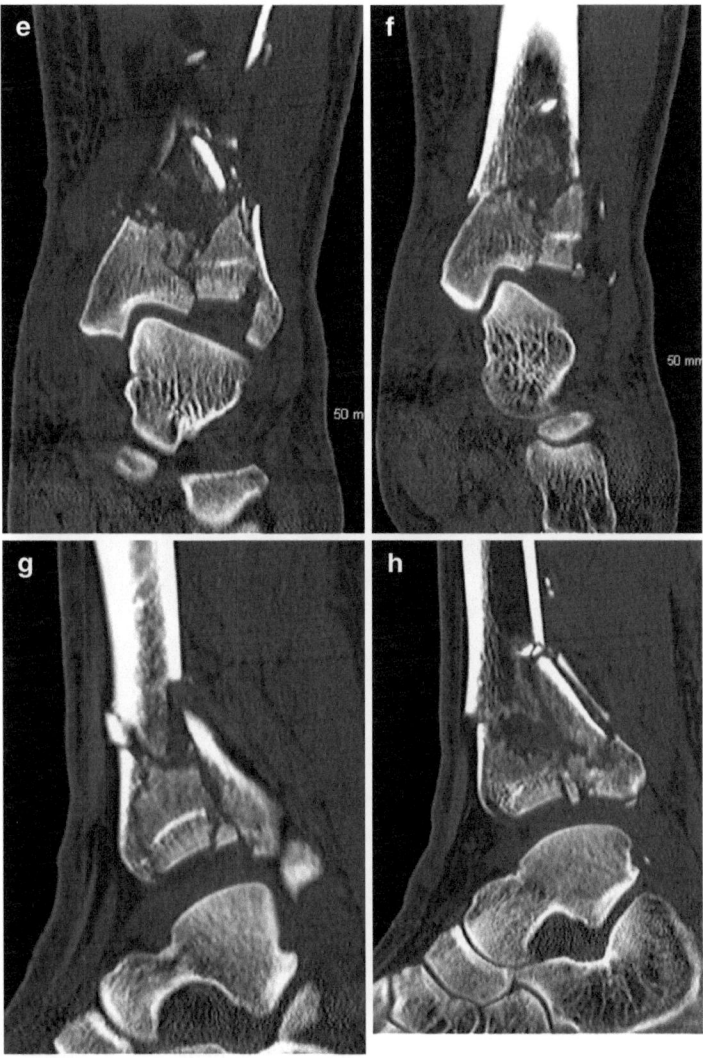

Fig. 17.3 (continued)

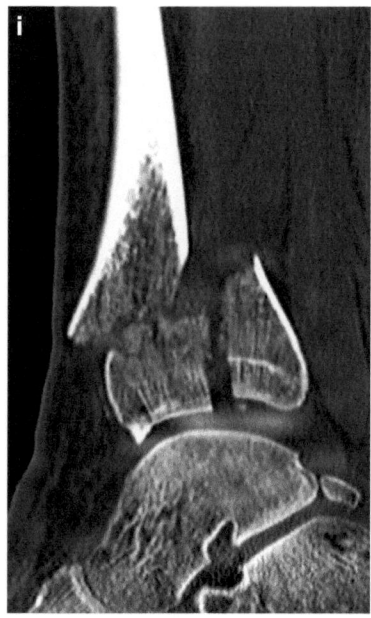

Fig. 17.3 (continued)

Fracture Reduction

Planning for definitive fixation began with placement of the external fixator. Tibial pins were placed outside of the zone of injury to avoid plate overlap, while the calcaneal pin was placed in the optimal position to use later as a distraction device for improved joint visualization, while avoiding creating an unbalanced dorsi- or plantarflexion moment. Fracture reduction and definitive fixation began with addressing the posterior half. Through the posterolateral approach, initial bridging fixation of the fibula was achieved with a metaphyseal locking compression plate. After restoring fibular length, the medial coronal split (Fig. 17.3i) was localized via fluoroscopy, and through a small posteromedial approach, the entrapped posterior tibialis tendon was identified and freed from the fracture site. Attention turned back to the posterolateral incision where posterior Volkmann fragments (Fig. 17.3a) and the medial column fragment were provisionally reduced and held with pointed reduction clamps and 0.062 Kirschner wires, respectively. After confirming adequate joint surface reduction via imaging, definitive fixation of the posterior reconstruction was held with an inverted four-hole proximal humerus plate (Fig. 17.4a–c). Using this plate in an inverted fashion allows one to achieve desired trajectory to capture fragments in a variety of angles. In this case, it allowed not only to hold the reduction of the posterolateral fragments, but also facilitated placement of a screw in an anteromedial trajectory to capture the medial column fragment. Care was taken to avoid placing fixation that would interfere with the patient's subsequent staged anterior surgery. After fixation of the posterior and medial fracture fragments, the patient was closed primarily and brought back 1 week later to address the anterior half of the fracture. With the fibular, posterior, and medial portions of the fracture fixed, this left only the anterolateral (Chaput) fragment left to reconstruct. Via an anterolateral approach, and using the external fixator as a distractor for direct visualization of the joint, articular surface reduction was obtained and held provisionally with 0.045 and 0.062 Kirschner wires. Confirming anatomic reduction of the articular surface, an anterolateral precontoured periarticular plate was placed with fixation initially placed distally. Following distal plate fixation, the metadiaphysis and length of the anterior tibia was restored and fixed proximally, in a bridge-like fashion. Confirming desired reduction and hardware position with fluoroscopy, the patient was closed primarily (Fig. 17.5a–c).

Postoperative Plan

A short leg splint was placed and replaced with a walking boot at the first postoperative visit (1 week). Posterolateral and anterolateral incisions were healed and sutures removed at approximately 3 weeks. The posteromedial incision sutures were removed at the 4-week follow-up timepoint. The patient was non-weight bearing for 3 months and gradually advanced. Ankle range of motion was begun upon final suture removals. Clinical and radiographic follow-up was done till union.

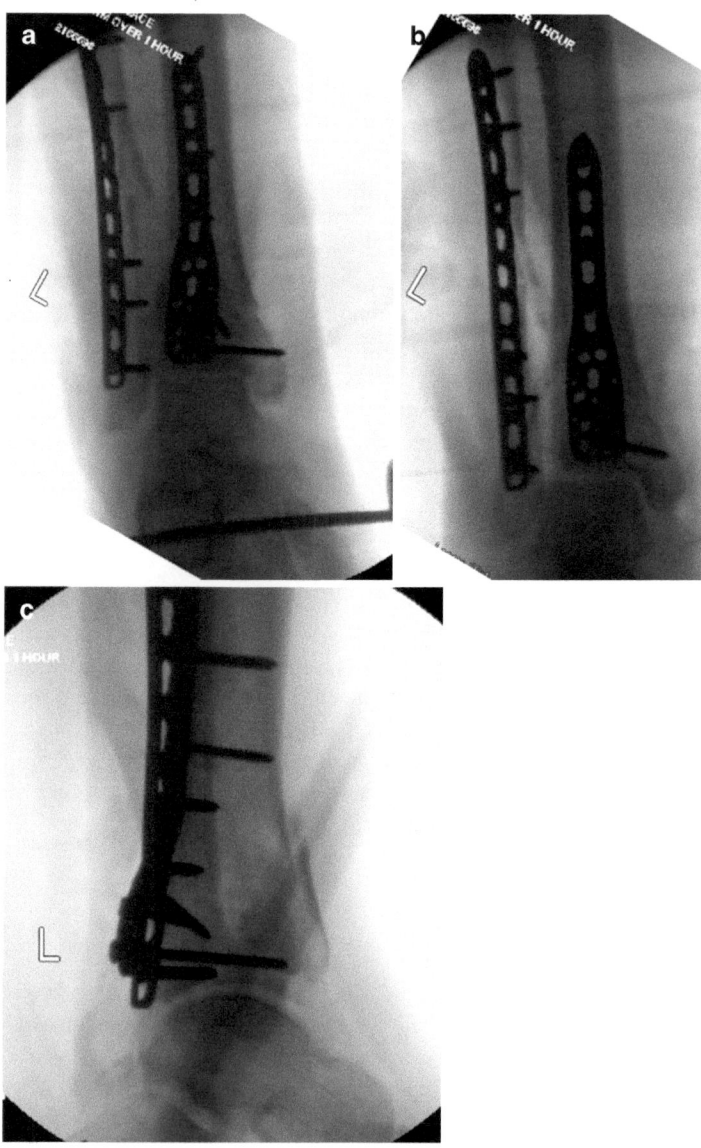

Fig. 17.4 (**a–c**) Initial portion of the definitive fixation restoring the Volkmann fragment and fibular length via the posterolateral approach. The patient remained in the external fixator and the anterior component was delayed in order to allow for the soft tissues to recover

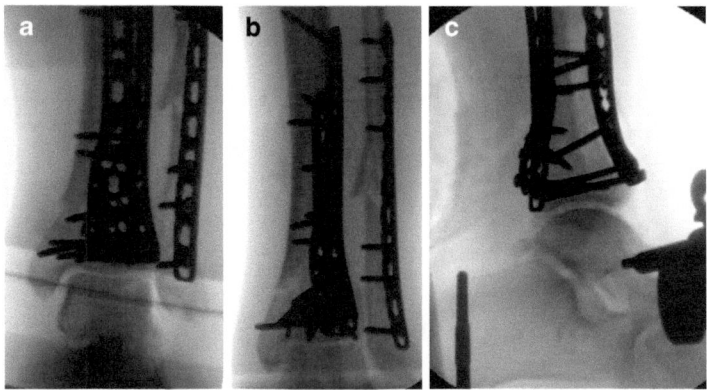

Fig. 17.5 (**a–c**) Definitive fixation of the anterior portion exhibiting restoration of the articular surface and balanced fixation that bridges the metaphyseal comminution

Outcome

Patient was made non-weight bearing for 3 months and subsequently advanced with maintained hardware position and callus formation. No joint line disruption or hardware migration was noted upon weight bearing and the patient healed uneventfully, reporting no pain with weight bearing, although reduced range of motion compared to the other side at 9 months follow-up (Fig. 17.6a–d). Radiographs at final follow-up note a healed fibular, tibial joint articular surface and metadiaphysis, despite a persistent loss of medial cortex, which was present on initial injury presentation.

Complications

None. No plans for hardware removal.

Salient Points/Pearls

- Respect the soft tissues. Delayed treatment in a splint or an external fixator should be employed liberally until swelling subsides [2, 5].

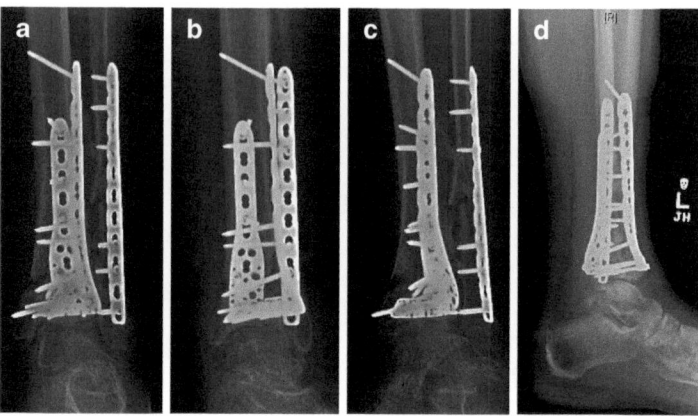

Fig. 17.6 (**a–d**) Radiographs at final follow-up exhibiting well healed pilon fracture with well maintained hardware. The patient reported no pain with weight bearing, although reported slightly decreased range of motion compared to the other side

- Dual incision approaches can help minimize soft tissue trauma by avoiding excessive retraction or stripping often needed with a single approach [2].
- Have a low threshold to stage and delay definitive fixation, and use multiple incisions to further protect and allow for soft tissue healing [2, 5].
- An appropriate skin bridge (5.9 cm) should be drawn out and marked on the skin to allow for predictable wound healing.
- Careful analysis of the CT scan can help dictate incision placement, but also help plan placement of provisional and definitive fixation. Also, note the possibility of soft tissue entrapment, especially posteromedially. Typically, this entrapped structure is the posterior tibialis tendon, but can often include the neurovascular bundle [1].
- Reconstructive goals can be simplified by converting the complex patterns into simpler fractures prior to ultimate definitive fixation. In this case, restore the classic fragments first (Volkmann, medial, and Chaput), then piece them back together. In other words, recreate the constant fragment

(Volkmann), fix it to the medial fragment, then restore the anterolateral fragment and fix it to the already fixed posteromedial portion [3, 4].

- Remember to address and buttress both the lateral and medial columns with plates that span and employ appropriate length.
- Density of fixation should be more rigid toward the articular surface with a less rigid fixation implemented as you move proximally toward the diaphysis to match the modulus of elasticity of bone.
- Patients should remain non-weight bearing for a minimum of 3 months and progress gradually.

References

1. Eastman JG, Firoozabadi R, Benirschke SK, Barei DP, Dunbar RP. Entrapped posteromedial structures in pilon fractures. J Orthop Trauma. 2014;28:528–33.
2. Liporace FA, Yoon RS. Decisions and staging leading to definitive open management of pilon fractures: where have we come from and where are we now? J Orthop Trauma. 2012;26:488–98.
3. Mehta S, Gardner MJ, Barei DP, Benirschke SK, Nork SE. Reduction strategies through the anterolateral exposure for fixation of type B and C pilon fractures. J Orthop Trauma. 2011;25:116–22.
4. Amorosa LF, Brown GD, Greisberg J. A surgical approach to posterior pilon fractures. J Orthop Trauma. 2010;24:188–93.
5. Sirkin M, Sanders R, DiPasquale T, Herscovici Jr D. A staged protocol for soft tissue management in the treatment of complex pilon fractures. J Orthop Trauma. 1999;13:78–84.

Chapter 18
Treatment of Pilon Fracture in External Fixator

Marilyn Heng, Michael J. Weaver, and Mitchel B. Harris

Clinical Scenario

A 79-year-old female sustained a mechanical trip down four steps resulting in immediate pain, swelling, and inability to bear weight on her left leg. She is a nonsmoker with a medical history significant only for hypertension. She first presented to the local emergency department where it was confirmed that she sustained an isolated left leg injury. X-rays revealed a left pilon fracture with shaft extension. She was transferred to the emergency department at our tertiary care center for definitive management.

On physical examination, the patient's ankle was swollen and ecchymotic with gross deformity and considerable tenderness to palpation. Her distal neurovascular examination was normal. Radiographs of the left ankle demonstrated a displaced intra-articular

M. Heng (✉)
Harvard Medical School Orthopaedic Trauma Initiative, Boston, MA, USA

Brigham and Women's Hospital, Department of Orthopaedics,
Boston, MA, USA

Massachusetts General Hospital, Department of Orthopaedics,
Boston, MA, USA
e-mail: mheng@mgh.harvard.edu

M.J. Weaver • M.B. Harris
Harvard Medical School Orthopaedic Trauma Initiative, Boston, MA, USA

Brigham and Women's Hospital, Department of Orthopaedics,
Boston, MA, USA

© Springer International Publishing Switzerland 2016   199
N.C. Tejwani (ed.), *Fractures of the Tibia: A Clinical Casebook*,
DOI 10.1007/978-3-319-21774-1_18

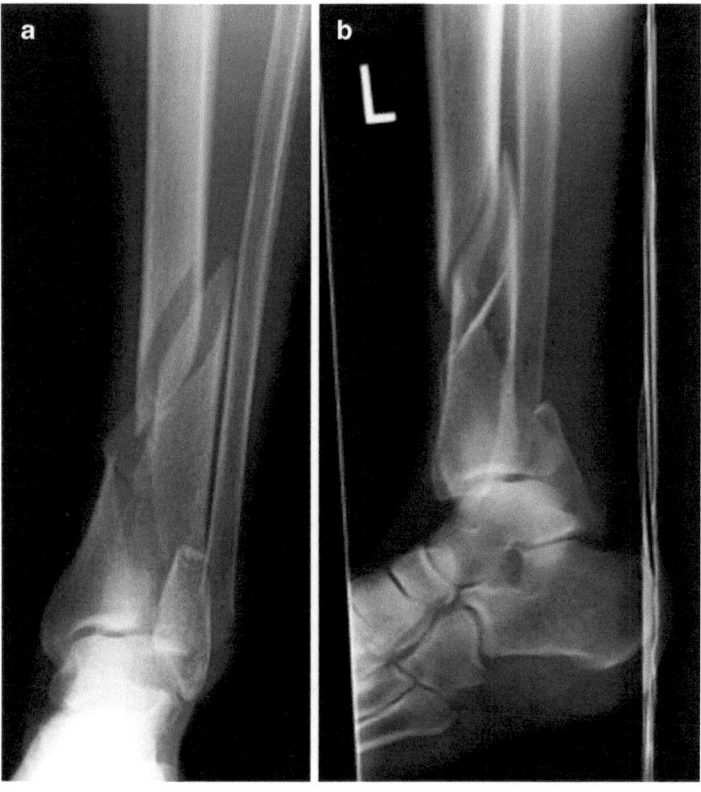

Fig. 18.1 Initial injury radiographs AP left tibia (**a**) and lateral of left ankle (**b**)

fracture of the left distal tibia with spiral extension up the diaphysis and an associated completely displaced short oblique fracture of the fibula (Fig. 18.1).

Treatment Considerations and Planning

After assessment, a closed reduction with sedation was attempted and the patient's leg was placed into a below knee plaster splint. Postreduction x-rays revealed the fracture remained significantly shortened with mild improvement in the reduction of the articular surface.

At this point in time, as is often the case with pilon fractures, the patient's soft tissues were deemed too swollen for acute open fixation [1, 2]. A staged approach with initial external fixation and delayed internal fixation was planned. The morning following her injury, the patient was taken to the operating room and her left tibia and ankle were placed into an external fixator utilizing a delta-frame construct (Fig. 18.6). The goals of the external fixator application were to restore length, rotation, and alignment to the limb and to reduce the tibiotalar joint subluxation. The restoration of length with the external fixator was especially evident in comparison of the state of the fibular fracture before and after external fixation (Fig. 18.2).

In order to obtain better images and information for definitive fracture management, a CT scan of the ankle should be performed after closed reduction and external fixation of a pilon fracture. The CT scan aids in further delineation of the fracture pattern at the articular surface. In our case, the intra-articular fracture pattern was relatively simple, consisting of one main sagittal fracture line and a small avulsion fracture off of the distal fibula (i.e., a Wagstaff fragment) (Fig. 18.3). The diaphyseal extension of the fracture was of a spiral nature with a large posterior butterfly-fragment.

Surgical Timing

Following external fixation and CT scan, the patient was discharged to a rehabilitation facility due to her advanced age and postoperative non-weight-bearing status. She was seen in follow-up 12 days post external fixation for clinical examination. At that time, the patient's soft tissue swelling had decreased significantly and the skin "wrinkle sign" was positive. However, the patient was a thin, elderly lady with very fragile, thin skin that was even more apparent now that her swelling had subsided. Follow-up x-rays demonstrated displacement of the diaphyseal component of the

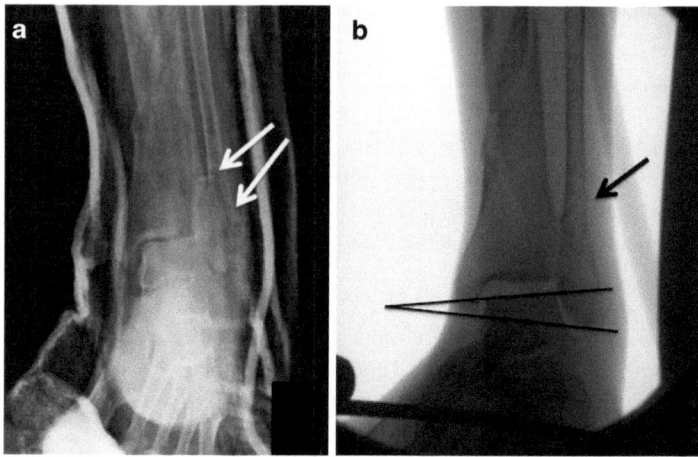

Fig. 18.2 Preexternal fixation radiograph demonstrating complete displacement of the fibular fracture; *white arrows* indicate fracture ends (**a**). Restoration of length demonstrated through reduction of the fibula fracture, *black arrow*, and restoration of talocrural angle, *black lines* (**b**)

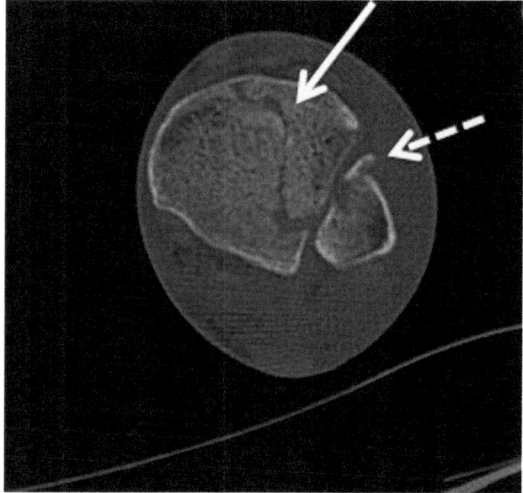

Fig. 18.3 Axial CT cut of tibial plafond demonstrating the main sagittal fracture line at the articular surface, *white solid arrow*, and of the Wagstaff avulsion fracture off the fibula, *white dashed arrow*

fracture, while the articular surface appeared well aligned. Given the patient's fragile skin and the concern that a formal open approach for internal fixation would predispose her to wound coverage and healing problems and recognizing the satisfactory alignment of the fracture in the external fixator, the decision was made to proceed with definitive treatment in the external fixator augmented with limited fixation with percutaneous screws.

Intraoperative Tips and Tricks for Reduction/Fixation

Use of CT Scan for Preoperative Planning of Lag Screws Perpendicular to Fracture Line

Careful examination of the CT scan is required to effectively plan the placement of percutaneous lag screws. The ideal placement of these screws is perpendicular to the plane of the fracture line. Fig. 18.4 demonstrates our preoperative plan of lag screws in order to compress across fracture lines at the articular surface and within the diaphysis.

Perfect Circle Technique for Percutaneous Lag Screws

Intraoperatively, in order to place screws perpendicular to the fracture line as preoperatively planned, we employed a "perfect-circle fluoroscopic technique." This technique is useful to "target" the lag screw based upon preoperative CT imaging and radiographic landmarks. A large C-arm image intensifier is utilized and is used to first image the fracture line across which the lag screw is to be placed. Either the C-arm or the limb is rotated until the beam of radiation is perpendicular to the fracture line – it is at this point that the fracture line on the fluoroscopic image will "disappear." The C-arm's position is locked in place. At the desired spot for the lag screw, a stab incision is made with the scalpel, a hemostat is used to spread down to bone, and a 3.5 mm drill guide is inserted onto the bone. The drill guide is manipulated until it is positioned with

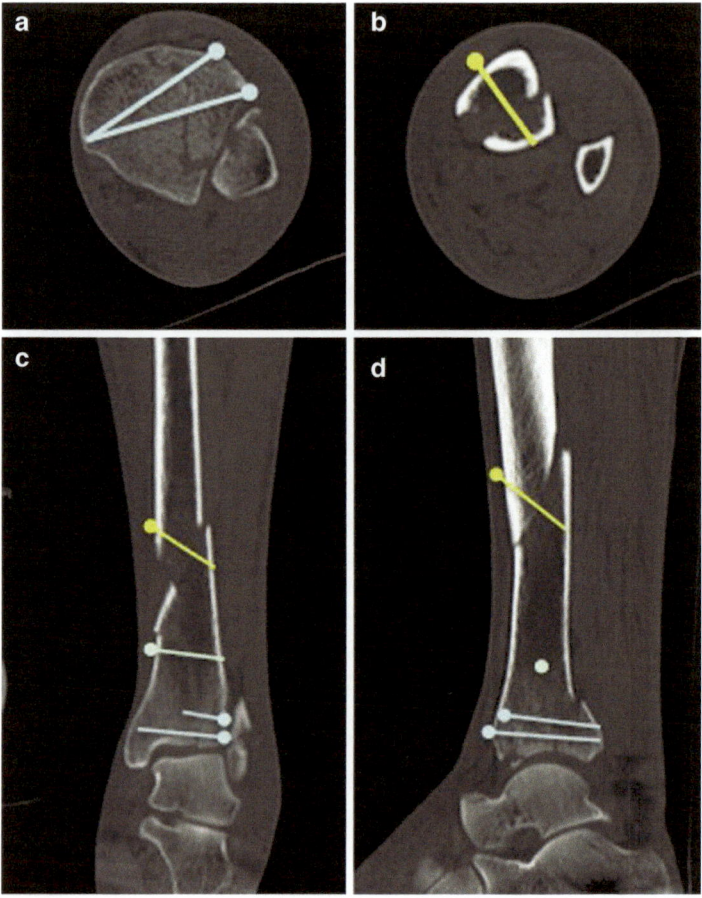

Fig. 18.4 Preoperative plan using CT scan for placement of percutaneous lag screws, *colored pinheads*. (**a**) Axial section at tibial plafond, (**b**) axial section at diaphyseal level, (**c**) coronal section of tibia, (**d**) sagittal section of tibia

a "perfect circle" on the fluoroscopic image, indicating that this trajectory is parallel to the C-arm beam and, hence, perpendicular to the fracture line (Fig. 18.5a, b). The drill guide is held in place and a 3.5 mm drill is drilled through the near cortex. A smooth 2.0 mm K-wire is placed through the drill guide to mark the site of the drill hole. The drill guide is then switched over the K-wire to

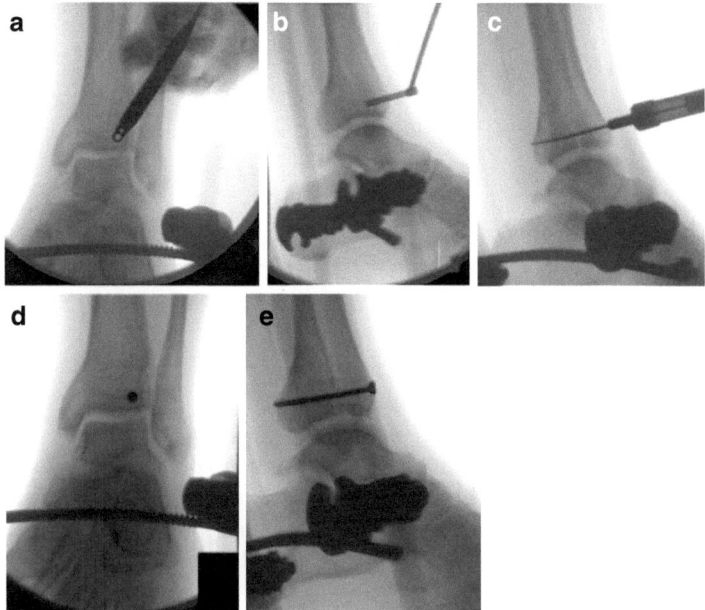

Fig. 18.5 Perfect circle technique for percutaneous lag screw insertion. Obtaining perfect circle with drill guide (**a, b**). Measurement and insertion of lag screw across articular fracture line (**c–e**) *Note: Fig.s shown are from a different case than the one presented in the text

the 2.5 mm drill guide. The K-wire is removed and the 2.5 mm drill is used to drill the far cortex. The screw length is measured and a 3.5 mm cortex screw is inserted, lagging the fracture in place (Fig. 18.5c–e). This technique is particularly useful near the ankle joint where precise screw placement is important to avoid penetrating the tibial plafond or distal tibiofibular joint.

Adjustment of Temporary External Fixator to Definitive Treatment Construct

The use of the external fixator for temporary vs. definitive treatment has different priorities and, hence, different principles. In converting our temporary external fixator to one for

Table 18.1 Methods to increase the stability of an external fixator

Use of additional pins
Use of additional bars
Placement of pins in different planes
Placement of bars in different planes
Decreased distance between bar and skin
Pin placement in a near-near, far-far fashion
Use of pins with larger diameter

definitive treatment, our goal for the construct changed to the requirement for greater stability and no longer required the consideration of keeping the fixator pins outside the area of future internal fixation. Additional Schanz pins were added to the construct near to the fracture site and the bars were positioned as close to the skin as possible now that the swelling in the limb was decreased. Table 18.1 outlines additional factors that will increase the stability of an external fixation construct.

Maintenance of Plantigrade Foot in External Fixator

When treating a fracture definitively in an external fixator, it is important to employ a strategy to prevent secondary equinus deformity. For temporary external fixation constructs, a padded footplate can be used (Fig. 18.6). However, in situations when the external fixator will be the definitive treatment and is expected to be in place for several months, the footplate can be bulky and cumbersome. For the purposes of definitive treatment in the external fixator, our preference is to utilize an additional pin in the external fixator construct that can be placed in the base of the 1st metatarsal, the talus, or as a second transcalcaneal pin. In our case, a pin into the talus was inserted (Fig. 18.7) in order to fix the hind foot in a plantigrade position.

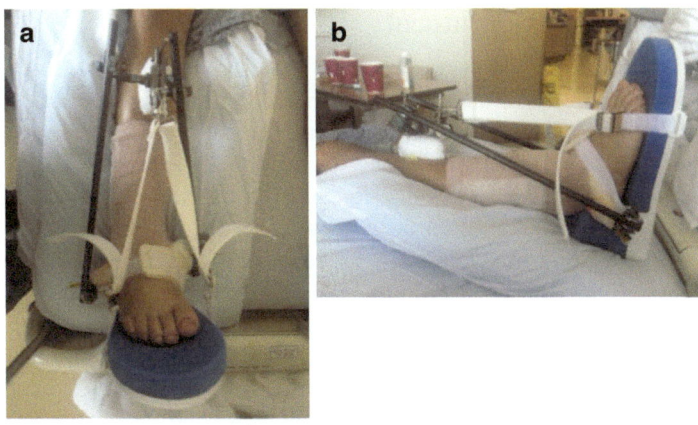

Fig. 18.6 Padded footplate to prevent equinus contracture. (**a**) Front view, (**b**) side view

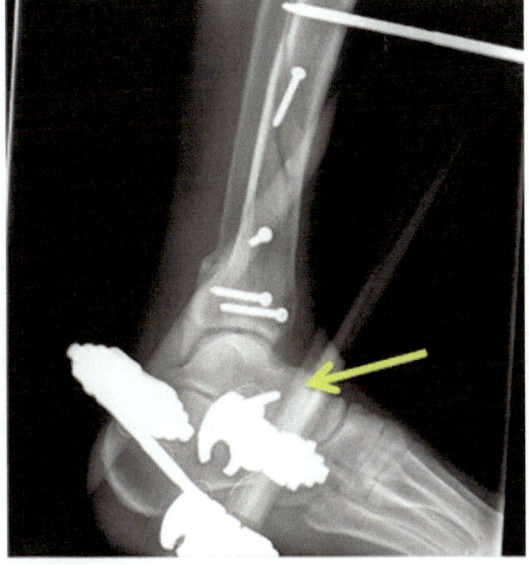

Fig. 18.7 External fixator with *talar pin*, *yellow arrow*, to fix the foot in a plantigrade position

Postoperative Protocol

Postoperatively, the patient was restricted to non-weight bearing on the operative leg. Pin sites were cleansed and dressed as per routine protocol. At 10 weeks status post application of the external fixator, x-rays exhibited good healing along the metaphyseal and epiphyseal fracture lines, with slower healing evident along the diaphysis.

The patient was consented for removal of the external fixator with fluoroscopic examination under anesthesia. Following removal of the external fixator, there was no gross motion at the diaphyseal fracture site or the intra-articular fracture site. The patient was placed into a short fiberglass walking cast and instructed to begin progression of weight bearing.

Two weeks following removal of the external fixator, the patient was transitioned into an Aircast boot and continued with physical therapy progressing to full weight bearing. Passive and active ankle range of motion (ROM) exercises were commenced. At 6 weeks following removal of the external fixator, the patient was instructed to begin weaning use of the Aircast boot and to continue working on ROM and progressive strengthening and proprioception of the ankle.

Follow-Up

Following removal of the external fixator, the patient was seen at regular intervals for approximately 4 months. By this time her fracture was completely united (Fig. 18.8). She had returned to weight bearing as tolerated in normal footwear and all of her activities as tolerated, including aerobics. Clinically, all pin sites were well healed and her ankle range of motion was from 15° dorsiflexion to 30° of plantarflexion and painless. The patient was discharged from regular follow-up.

Salient Points/Pearls

- Distal tibia fractures with articular extension can be definitively treated in an external fixation, especially with actual or potential soft tissue compromise.

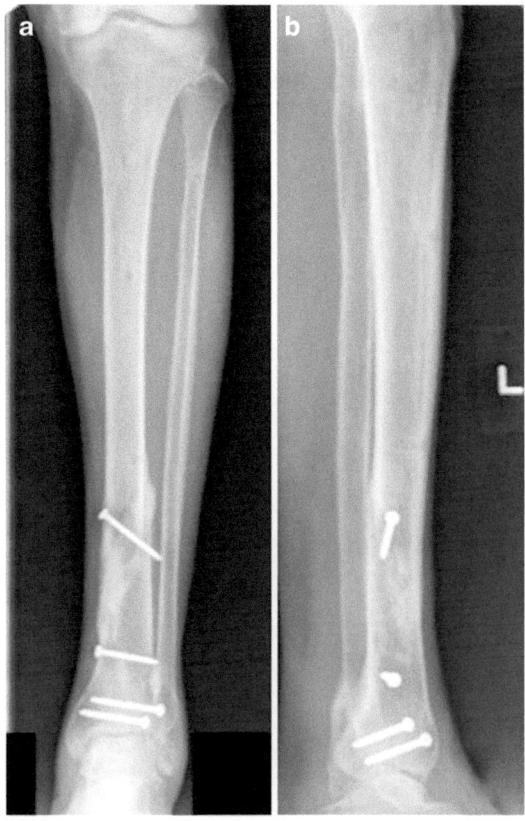

Fig. 18.8 Follow-up radiographs at 4 months status post removal of the external fixator demonstrating union of the fracture, (**a**) AP view, (**b**) lateral view

- The articular surface must be reduced and fixed securely. Use of the perfect circle technique with fluoroscopy is recommended to insert screws perpendicular to the fracture plane.
- External fixation principles must be followed to allow for increased stability and holding the ankle and foot in neutral position.
- Weight bearing is restricted until bony healing is evident.

References

1. Sirkin M, Sanders R, DiPasquale T, Herscovici D. A staged protocol for soft tissue management in the treatment of complex pilon fractures. J Orthop Trauma. 1999;13(2):78–84.
2. Rammelt S, Endres T, Grass R, Zwipp H. The role of external fixation in acute ankle trauma. Foot Ankle Clin. 2004;9(3):455–74.

Chapter 19
Distal Tibia Pilon: Staged Fixation – Fibula Fixation and then Tibia

Aaron T. Creek and Kyle J. Jeray

Case Presentation

This is a 45-year old maintenance worker who fell from scaffolding and sustained a closed right pilon fracture. Figure 19.1 represents the acute injury. He was initially seen at an outside hospital where a trauma evaluation was performed. The isolated orthopedic injury described was identified, and spanning external fixation was applied that day to the right lower extremity. The following day the patient was transferred to our level one trauma hospital for continued management. Upon presentation, the patient had no sensory or motor deficits and had a normal vascular exam. He had significant swelling of the right ankle with early fracture blisters on the medial aspect of the ankle. The external fixation was noted to be loose and adequate length and alignment was not restored.

A.T. Creek, MD • K.J. Jeray, MD (✉)
Department of Orthopaedic Surgery, Greenville Health System,
Greenville, SC, USA
e-mail: kjeray@ghs.org

© Springer International Publishing Switzerland 2016 211
N.C. Tejwani (ed.), *Fractures of the Tibia: A Clinical Casebook*,
DOI 10.1007/978-3-319-21774-1_19

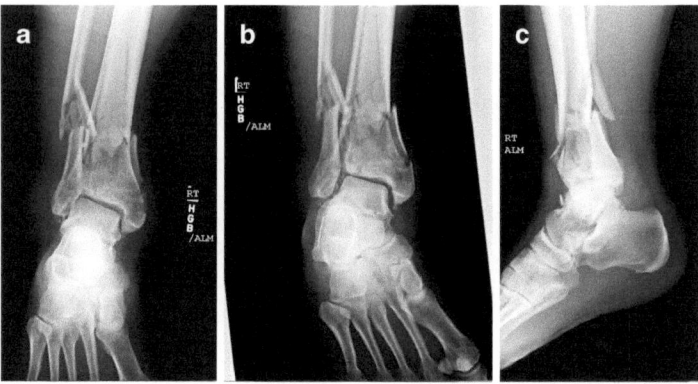

Fig. 19.1 Injury films showing the fractured tibial plafond with comminuted fibula fracture on (**a**) AP, (**b**) oblique, and (**c**) lateral projections. Notice the slight valgus angulation due to the compromised lateral column

Initial Treatment and Timing of Surgery

The following day, revision of the temporary external fixator and plating of the fibula was done to restore length and overall alignment.

Surgical Tact

Position

Supine with foam rectangle to elevate limb to allow for unobstructed lateral c-arm image.

Approach

Direct lateral to expose fibula recognizing that there needs to be adequate spacing of at least 5–6 cm for additional surgical incisions to fix the tibia.

Fracture Reduction and Closure

The degree of comminution makes absolute stability of the fibula impossible so relative length and stability was the goal. A 12-hole distal fibula locking plate was placed spanning the fracture and was secured proximally with two screws. The fracture was pulled out to length as judged by the relative alignment of the comminuted fibular fragments and was secured distally with a unicortical screw. Adjustments were made to obtain the best reduction possible and then appropriate screw fixation was made both proximal and distal to the fracture. During the plating of the fibula, while the lateral structures were exposed, the peroneal retinaculum and lateral ligaments were noted to be disrupted and were repaired

Figure 19.2 shows the injury following temporary spanning external fixation with the fibula plated. The fibular plating provided added stability to the lateral column and aided in restoring lateral column length. Many of the opinions concerning fibular reduction and fixation in pilon fractures are direct extensions of Rüedi and Allgöwer's original principles on open reduction and

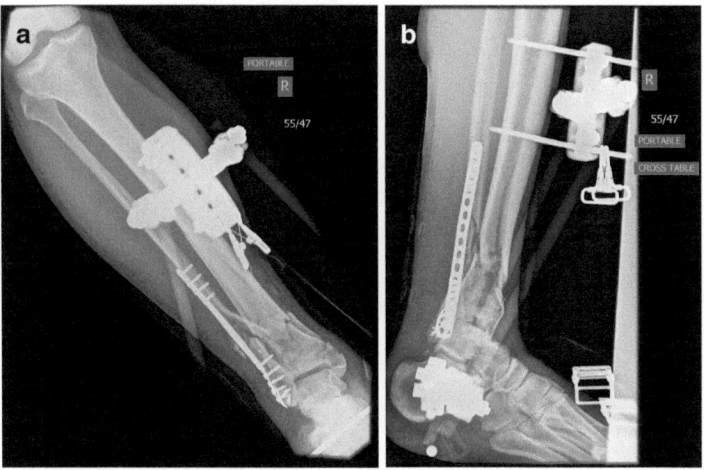

Fig. 19.2 Postoperative films after limited ORIF of the fibula and spanning external fixation of the ankle as shown on (**a**) AP and (**b**) lateral projections

internal fixation (ORIF) of pilon fractures [4]. They identified four technical principles in pilon ORIF: reduction and stabilization of the fibula fracture, anatomic restoration of the tibial articular surface, support of the impacted articular surface with bone graft, and buttress support of the medial tibia to prevent varus angulation. These authors recognized that the fixed fibula could serve as a guide for appropriate length and alignment of the tibia through restoration of the lateral column as well as serving to correct the valgus deformity of the distal tibia if one exists on injury. They found that this technique can also indirectly reduce the anterolateral and posterior tibial fracture fragments through ligamentotaxis.

As the skin blisters were significant on the medial and anterior ankle, delayed fixation of the pilon was planned. Staged fixation of pilon fractures, once heavily debated, has essentially become the standard of care in pilon fracture management. Staged fixation allows the surgeon to potentially avoid soft tissue complications, reduce infection rates, thus improving overall outcomes ([3, 4, 6, 8].

After a 3-day admission for pain control and physical therapy for crutch training, our patient was discharged from the hospital and kept non-weight bearing on his right lower extremity.

Definitive Treatment

This gentleman returned to clinic 2 weeks from the index procedure and there was noted wrinkling of his skin and resolution of his bloody fracture blisters. He then returned to the operating room that week and underwent right distal tibia ORIF.

Surgical Tact

Position

Supine with foam rectangle to elevate limb to allow for unobstructed lateral c-arm image.

Approach

Anterior approach with anterior periarticular plate.

Fracture Reduction and Closure

The bulk of the reduction is obtained indirectly early with external fixation and plating of the fibula as demonstrated by the postspanning external fixation computed tomography (CT) scan (Fig. 19.3). The remainder of the reduction is done under direct visualization primarily addressing the articular fragments using intraoperative distraction with the external fixator or a femoral distractor placed intraoperatively. Based on the CT scan, the approach along with

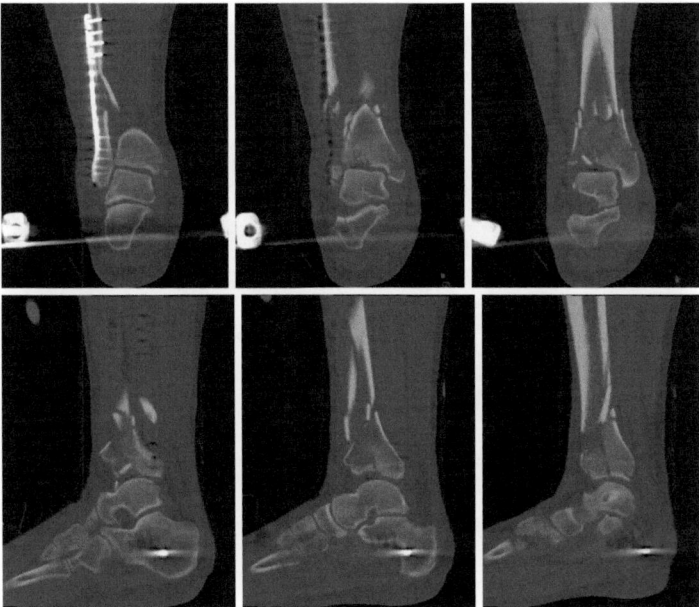

Fig. 19.3 Representative CT images of the pilon injury status post fibula ORIF and ankle spanning fixation showing the reduction that is possible with lateral column stabilization and ankle ligamentotaxis

the position and placement of the screws were preoperatively planned. In this case, it was determined that the fracture could be reduced through a single anterior approach and anterolateral plating. The plan was to lag the long, spiral shaft fracture; plate the injury anteriorly; and not address the seemingly stable medial malleolus unless it displaced intraoperatively.

No tourniquet was used based on our personal preference. If substantial bleeding is encountered, a tourniquet can safely be used. Closure was done with monocryl in the subcutaneous tissue and a running nylon stitch for the skin. We prefer a running stitch in the skin to keep handling of the skin to a minimum. A bulky posterior splint was applied. Figure 19.4 shows the postoperative radiographs with the definitive fixation.

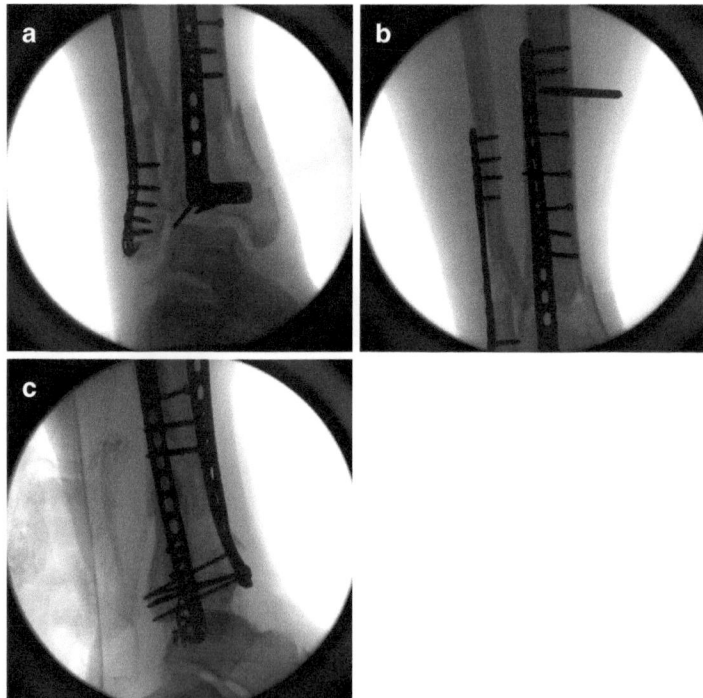

Fig. 19.4 Intraoperative films showing definitive fixation in (**a**, **b**) AP and (**c**, **d**) lateral projections. Multiple fluoroscopy images were taken intraoperatively to show that the distal and lateral most tibial-plate screw was extra-articular

Postoperative Plan

The patient had the splint changed on postoperative day 2 prior to discharge. The patient was instructed to be non-weight bearing on that extremity.

At the 2-week follow up, there were no issues with wound healing. The sutures were removed and a short leg fiberglass cast was applied for 4 weeks. At 6 weeks from definitive surgery, the cast was removed, another wound check was performed, and range of motion exercises started. He was placed in a walker boot to allow protection of the foot/ankle, to keep the foot out of equinus, and to allow the mode of immobilization to be removed for range of motion exercises. The patient was kept non-weight bearing even though the boot was in place for an additional 6 weeks.

Outcome

At 3 months, weight bearing was initiated after radiographs confirmed adequate healing. At a little more than 4 months, he was complaining of some ankle stiffness but was overall doing well and ambulating in his work boot. At 7 months, he was back to regular, floor-level duties at work, and at 1 year he was back to climbing ladders and had only occasional ankle swelling. Figure 19.5 shows radiographs at 6 months and 12 months postoperative.

Salient Points/Pearls/Tips and Tricks

- Initial Evaluation: The first consideration in the treatment of pilon fractures is the overall health of the patient. Patients that have pilon injuries are often victims of high-energy trauma and have multiple other injuries or may have other health concerns that increase the surgical risks to the patient. In these cases, it is important to consult with appropriate trauma or hospitalist services to evaluate the overall health of the patient and the risks and benefits of the treatment options. Once the patient is cleared for surgery, the planning process for fixation strategies begins.

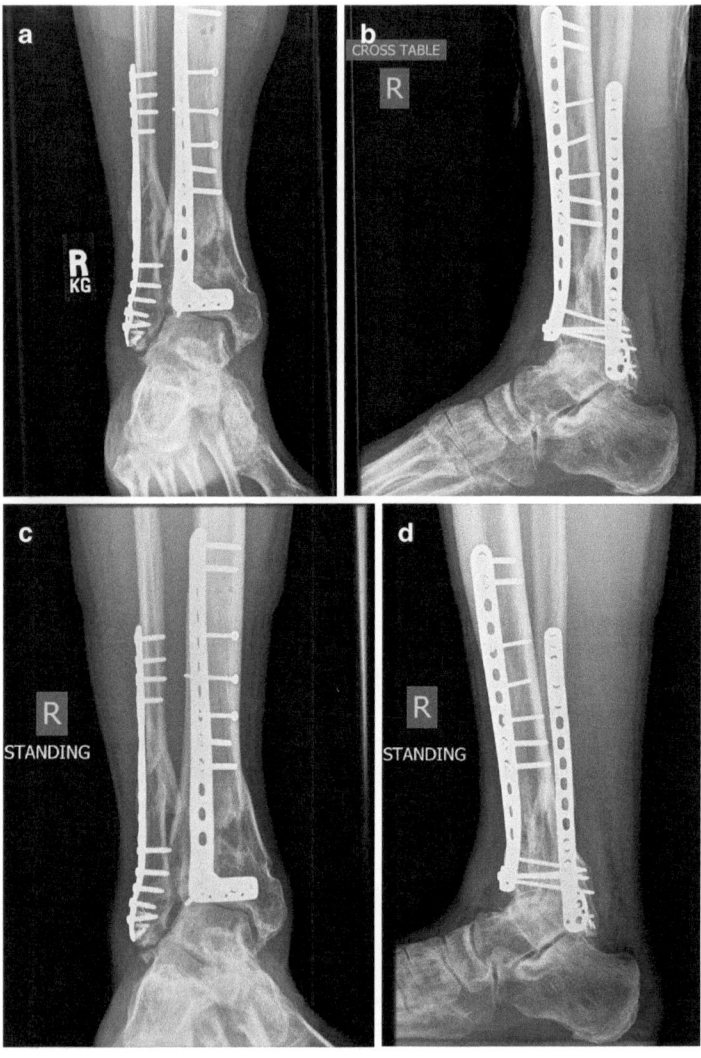

Fig. 19.5 Healed tibial plafond fracture at 6 months on the (**a**) AP and (**b**) lateral projections and again at 12 months with (**c**) AP and (**d**) lateral projections. There is some evidence of early ankle arthrosis, as is expected with this injury

- Spanning external fixation with acute fibula plating: As discussed above in Reudi and Allgower's basic principles of pilon management, obtaining length of the lateral column is of utmost importance. One way to do this is by addressing the fibula fracture with ORIF when placing the spanning external fixator. In 1998, Williams et al. [7] published their experience with plating the fibula early in a retrospective clinical study. Seven of the 22 patients had complications related to plating of the fibula, including five infections and two nonunions. Three of the four surgeons participating in that study no longer routinely plate the fibula. Two other studies published in the late 1990s presented different results from acute plating of the fibula and spanning external fixation. Sirkin et al. described only five partial thickness and two deep wound complications in their series of 56 patients. These instances were treated with local wound care and oral antibiotics, while Patterson et al. had no infections or soft tissue complications in their 21 patient series. Both studies included both open and closed fractures in their analysis [3, 6].
- While we do not routinely fix the fibula in all pilon fractures, we think that there are occasions where early fibular plating is beneficial. If the fibula is significantly shortened and appears to be amenable to either anatomic reduction or bridge plating, we advocate early fixation if length, alignment, and stability can be improved. Early fixation can also be helpful in restoring anatomic length of the overall injury when the distal tibia is comminuted and shortened such that it would be difficult to judge appropriate length with a spanning fixator. By fixing the lateral column anatomically there is no doubt that length has been restored to the overall construct and any residual varus must be coming from malreduction of the tibia, which can often be addressed with the external fixation.
- Pre-op planning: In the case that was presented here, the patient was initially seen at an outside facility and then transferred to us for definitive management. Many times the spanning fixation with or without the fibular plating is done at the transferring institution. We recommend that the surgeon who initially treats the fracture only span the ankle joint with external fixation

and refrain from fixing the fibula if he/she is not going to be the surgeon who addresses the definitive fixation. Thus, by avoiding acute fibular fixation, the definitive treatment plan is not compromised with a poorly placed fibular incision, or, worse yet, a poorly reduced and fixed (and often short) fibula fracture. Generally, the orthopedic trauma surgeon who will be performing the definitive ORIF can, for example, place the fibula incision posterior enough to allow for a future anterolateral incision or allow for reaccess through the posterior incision to fix a posterolateral fracture of the tibial plafond.

- Pin placement: Placement of the external fixation pins is also important in relation to the planned surgical approach and definitive fixation. The external fixator pins should be kept out of the zone of injury and away from planned approaches for definitive ORIF. Shah et al. describe a 24 % incidence of deep infection in cases in which the plate for definitive fixation covers a pin tract from initial spanning fixation, whereas in cases with no overlap the deep infection rate was 10 % [5]. This shows the importance of respecting the soft tissue injury and the eventual footprint of the plate used for definitive fixation in an effort to minimize postoperative infection. Close examination of our postoperative imaging in Fig. 19.4 above shows that we did not follow this recommendation in our example patient. Unfortunately, since the external fixation was placed by someone other than the surgeon responsible for the definitive fixation, we did not have control of how the external fixator pins were placed. Ideally we would have avoided placing it in the zone of injury as well as assuring that our fixation would not overlap pin sites to diminish the risk for infection.

- CT scans: In an effort to delineate the fracture pattern in pilon fractures, a computed tomography (CT) evaluation should be done. The CT scan should be obtained after spanning fixation to show the location of the fracture fragments and the extent of reduction obtained from ligamentotaxis and restoration of length (Fig. 19.3). This allows the surgeon to more accurately preoperatively plan the surgical approach and appropriately select the fixation strategy. Often times multiple small plates can be used through more than one incision to obtain a more satisfying reduction than just relying on the standard, often extensile, approach to the tibial plafond.

- Surgical approach: The surgical approach must be chosen based on fracture pattern and soft tissue injury. We suggest drawing out the intended incisions for ORIF of the distal tibia to ensure that there is at least 5–7 cm of skin-bridge between the fibula incision and the chosen tibial incision(s) if possible. Common teaching is that this technique prevents vascular compromise of the interposed flap. The idea of an adequate skin bridge was developed in the days when pilons were being fixed very soon after injury. Now that a staged procedure is favored, there is evidence that incisions can be closer together than originally taught as long as the surgeon considers the orientation of the incision in relation to vascular structures [1].

- Timing of fixation and the soft tissues: Timing of pilon ORIF is of utmost importance. A large body of literature exists concerning timing of pilon ORIF [8] report a 50 % decrease in wound complications with staged treatment after initial spanning fixation. Other studies have found similar results in regards to complications with early definitive treatment and also found that most pilon fractures treated with initial spanning fixation are ready for definitive ORIF between 7 and 21 days from the date of injury [3, 6].

- Improving visualization: To aid in the visualization and direct reduction of the intra-articular fracture beyond the typical distraction through the tibio-calcaneal fixator, sometimes adding a pin in the talar neck intraoperatively, and distracting through the tibio-talar pins allows for additive distraction directly at the involved joint improving visualization.

- Outcomes: Because they have an intra-articular injury in a weight bearing joint, even patients with an anatomic fracture reduction are at an increased risk for osteoarthritis compared to the general population. In 2003, Marsh et al. [2] describes worse function and higher incidence of osteoarthritis compared to controls at 5–11 years postoperative, but most patients were still satisfied with their results and the arthrodesis rate was only 5.4 % Therefore, it is important to educate the patient on the risks of osteoarthritis and future implications.

References

1. Howard JL. A prospective study evaluating incision placement and wound healing for tibial plafond fractures. J Orthop Trauma. 2008;22(5):299–305.
2. Marsh JL, Weigel DP, Dirschl DR. Tibial plafond fractures. How do these ankles function over time? J Bone Joint Surg Am. 2003;85-A(2):287–95.
3. Patterson M, Cole J. Two-staged delayed open reduction and internal fixation of severe pilon fractures. J Orthop Trauma. 1999;13(2):85–91.
4. Rüedi T, Allgöwer M. Fracures of the lower end of the tibia into the ankle joint: results 9 years after open reduction and internal fixation. Injury. 1969;1:92–9.
5. Shah CM, Babb PE, McAndrew CM, Brimmo O, Badarudeen S, Tornetta 3rd P, Ricci WM, Gardner MJ. Definitive plates overlapping provisional external fixator pin sites: is the infection risk increased? J Orthop Trauma. 2014;28(9):518–22.
6. Sirkin M, Sanders R, DiPasquale T, Herscovici Jr D. A staged protocol for soft tissue management in the treatment of complex pilon fractures. J Orthop Trauma. 1999;13(2):78–84.
7. Williams TM, Marsh JL. External fixation of tibial plafond fractures: is routine plating of the fibula necessary? J Orthop Trauma. 1998;12(1):16–20.
8. Wyrsch B, McFerran M, McAndrew M, Limbird T, Harper M, Johnson K, Schwartz H. Operative treatment of fractures of the tibial plafond. A randomized, prospective study. J Bone Joint Surg Am. 1996;78(11):1646–57.

Part V
Treatment of Non Union and Mal-Union of Tibia Fractures

Chapter 20
Nonunion Tibia Shaft Treated with IMN/Bone Grafting

Akhil Ashok Tawari, Harish Kempegowda, and Daniel S. Horwitz

Clinical Scenario

A 50-year-old gentleman presented with pain in his left tibia-fibula. He had sustained a closed segmental tibia-fibula fracture (Fig. 20.1a, b) following a motor vehicular accident one and a half years ago and had undergone open reduction and internal fixation with a reamed statically locked intramedullary nail for the tibia and plate osteosynthesis for the fibula. On presentation, he complained of 8/10 pain in the lower third tibia and anteriorly at the site of the distal interlocks that was aggravated with weight bearing. He also complained of frequent cramps in his left calf. He denied fever, chills or drainage from left lower extremity. He was nondiabetic, nonsmoker, and denied any other significant past medical or surgical illnesses. A focused clinical examination of the left lower extremity documented 10° diminished knee flexion and ankle dorsiflexion. He had multiple surgical scars that had healed with primary intention with no draining sinus or soft tissue compromise. The overlying skin seemed supple without any adhesions to the underneath structures. He had tenderness anteriorly

A.A. Tawari, MD • H. Kempegowda, MD • D.S. Horwitz, MD (✉)
Department of Orthopaedic Surgery, Geisinger Medical Center,
Danville, PA, USA
e-mail: dshorwitz@geisinger.edu

© Springer International Publishing Switzerland 2016   225
N.C. Tejwani (ed.), *Fractures of the Tibia: A Clinical Casebook*,
DOI 10.1007/978-3-319-21774-1_20

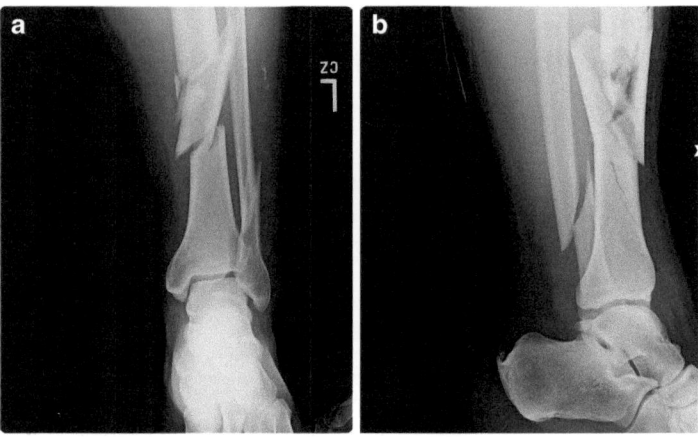

Fig. 20.1 (**a**, **b**) Antero-posterior (AP) and lateral radiographic images after sustaining trauma showing segmental fracture of the tibia and spiral fracture of the fibula at distal 1/3rd portion

over the fracture site and over the distal interlocking screws. He had normal capillary refill bilaterally with no motor or sensory deficits in his left lower extremity.

Treatment Considerations/Planning/Tests

A comprehensive radiological and hematological evaluation is mandatory in the management of nonunions as multiple risk factors are associated with impaired fracture healing. They can be patient related (age, comorbidities, tobacco, NSAIDS, and smoking), fracture related (open, segmental, comminuted, and articular), treatment related (quality of fracture reduction, soft tissue handling, and stabilization), and can be complicated by the presence of infection [1]. Radiological examination includes full length antero-posterior and lateral images of the tibia-fibula including the knee and the ankle. A bilateral standing long radiograph from the hips to the ankles must be obtained in the presence of angular deformities in the sagittal and coronal planes. CT scans with 3-D reconstruction and sagittal subtraction can be used when felt to be necessary. A "Gunsight" CT scan is useful in presence of a rotational deformity [2]. A standing lower extremity scanogram is desirable if significant limb length discrepancy exists. The hematological evaluation consists of a full metabolic profile (C.B.C, vitamin-D, glucose, thyroid profile, parathyroid profile, calcium, phosphorus, liver function test, and renal function test) and the tests to rule out infection ("C" reactive protein and erythrocyte sedimentation rate).

The radiological images of the patient revealed a segmental tibia fracture fixed with intramedullary interlocked nail and minimal callus (Fig. 20.2a, b). The intermediate fragment was angulated and healed to the distal fragment. The overall alignment of the proximal and the distal fragment was deemed acceptable as there was only a marginal angular deformity (valgus) and no rotational abnormality. On the lateral view, there was clear evidence of incomplete bridging in the anterior cortex. Although there was a suggestion of possible posterior bridging, it was partially obscured by the fibular plate. The length of the fibula was felt to have been

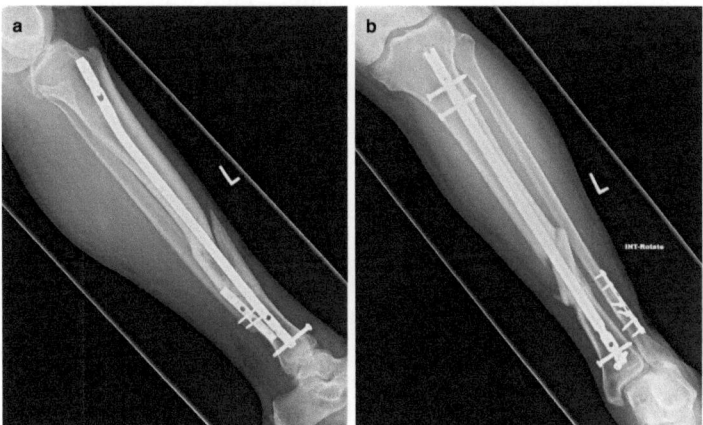

Fig. 20.2 (a, b) AP and lateral radiographic images at the time of presentation to us (one and a half years after the primary procedure). Minimal callus, statically locked intramedullary nail in the tibia and fracture gap in the anterior cortex can be appreciated

restored. A fine-cut CT scan was obtained, confirming the diagnosis of the nonunion (Fig. 20.3). The hematological investigations including tests for infection were within normal range. Thus, it was felt that the patient represented an aseptic, atrophic nonunion of the tibial shaft.

The principles of management of an aseptic atrophic nonunion include debridement of the nonunion site, stimulating the healing process, filling the bone defect (if any), minimizing fracture gap, and providing a stable fixation [3]. The available options in presence of an interlocking nail are isolated bone grafting, removal of the nail and application of a ring fixator, exchange nailing with bone grafting, nail removal with compression plating and bone grafting, nail retention/dynamization with compression plating and bone grafting, and the possible addition of a fibular osteotomy to any of these procedures in order to increase compression at the nonunion site [4].

The use of a ring fixator is preferable in presence of infection and massive deformity/segmental bone defect that may require bone transport. Plate fixation can achieve compression at the fracture site but requires extensive soft tissue dissection and periosteal stripping. In addition, plates are load-bearing devices and, hence, more prone to failure if the patient bears weight with persistent delayed union or nonunion. On the other hand, nails may be biomechanically preferred over plates, they require less soft tissue dissection during insertion and the endosteal reaming for the canal preparation may stimulate fracture healing [5–7, 8].

The potential addition of a fibular osteotomy in order to allow more compression at the nonunion site should be carefully considered. If it is felt that the fibular length will prevent tibial compression or only permit it by creating a varus deformity, then it is essential that the fibula is addressed in some way, with either a segmental resection or an oblique osteotomy.

Based on all these factors, the decision was made to proceed with exchange nailing utilizing a larger diameter nail and open bone grafting of the anterior defect as it was felt that compression would not close the gap completely.

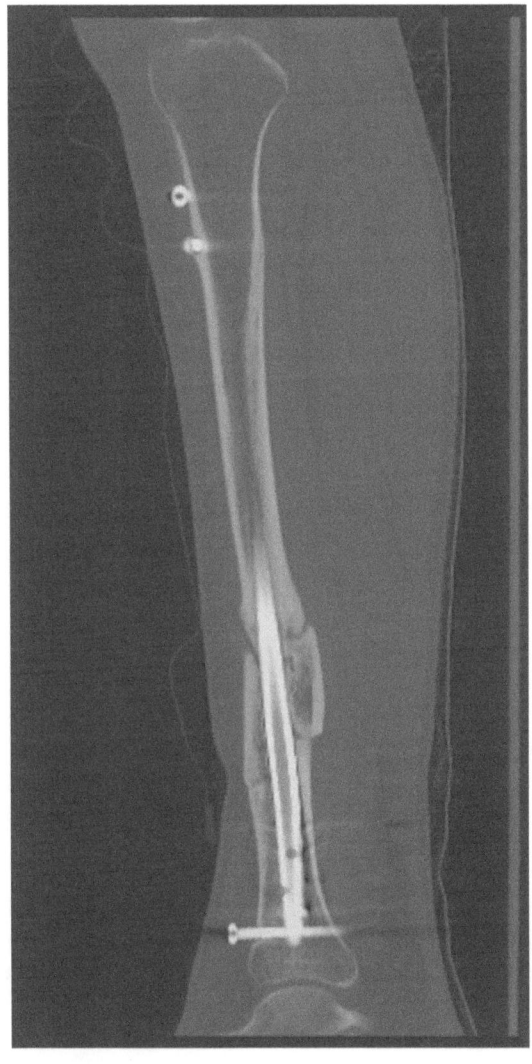

Fig. 20.3 CT image clearly displaying atrophic nonunion of the tibia, both anterior and posterior to the nail

Timing of Surgery

Fracture nonunion is a known complication of a segmental tibia fracture. Classically nonunion is defined when there is incomplete fracture healing within 9 months following injury along with no progression toward healing on serial radiographs for 3 consecutive months [9]. The timing of any surgical intervention depends upon the personality of the fracture, extent of healing, time since primary operation, and symptoms of the patient.

In this case, as the patient was still symptomatic one and a half years after his primary procedure and had clinical and radiological signs of nonunion, a decision was made to intervene once all the relevant tests were completed.

Intraoperative Tips and Tricks for Reduction/ Fixation

The procedure was performed in the supine position with the entire left lower extremity including the ipsilateral iliac crest prepped and draped. Proximal and distal interlocking screws were removed. An incision was then made over the patellar tendon, carried down through subcutaneous tissues and the patellar tendon to visualize the proximal aspect of the tibia nail. This surgical approach of the proximal nail (patellar splitting) followed the primary approach.

At this point, debridement at the nonunion site was carried out with the primary nail in place as the debridement can result in scratching/weakening of the nail. The nonunion site was exposed laterally raising full thickness flaps. A series of rongeur and curets were then used to remove all the interposed fibrous tissue anteriorly, medially, and laterally, and multiple specimens were sent for culture. The nail (10 mm) was removed and a ball tipped guide wire was placed into the canal. Sequential reaming of the tibia was done up to and including a 13.5 mm reamer and the reaming specimens were sent for culture as well. This was followed by harvesting of cancellous bone graft from the proximal tibia utilizing a small pituitary rongeur. A 12 mm nail was selected and fully seated down into the tibia. Two distal interlocks were placed in the standard freehand technique taking care that the new interlock holes did not match the primary ones. A dynamic proximal interlock was placed, and the compression device was used to provide compression at the nonunion site. This was followed by placement of the static proximal interlock. Approximately 8 cc of bone marrow was aspirated from the iliac crest and combined with 10 cc of cancellous allograft and 10 cc of proximal tibia autograft. This graft was placed into the nonunion site laterally and anteriorly (Fig. 20.4a, b), taking care to avoid over packing the anterior aspect as that can cause tension on the suture lines and impede wound healing possibly leading to wound drainage and infection.

Postoperative Protocols

The postoperative weight-bearing protocol is determined by the type of implant utilized. In general, intramedullary nails and ring fixators allow immediate full weight bearing as opposed to plates.

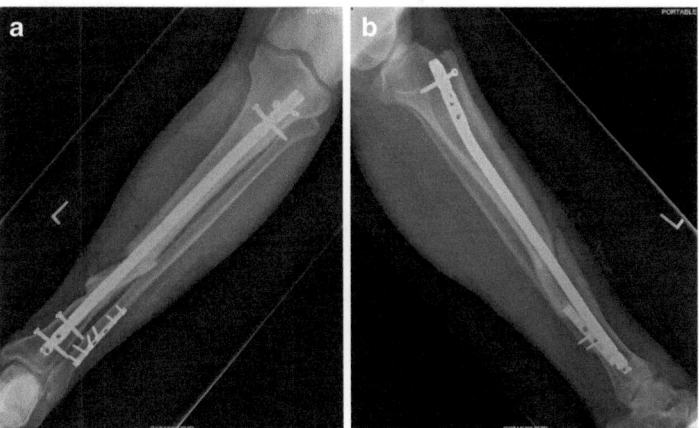

Fig. 20.4 (a, b) Immediate postoperative AP and lateral radiographic images showing larger diameter dynamically locked intramedullary nail and bone graft in the nonunion site

Splints/braces may be used to further augment the stability of fixation especially after application of plates. It is imperative to start the patients on aggressive physical therapy regimen stressing early range of motion. Patients should be counseled against using nicotine, and NSAIDS are best avoided [10].

Postoperatively this patient was started on aerobic conditioning and immediate weight bearing as tolerated. He underwent active and assisted range of motion of the hip, knee, and the ankle as well as gastrocnemius stretching exercises.

Follow-Up

Patients undergoing revision surgery for tibial nonunion [especially infected nonunions] are more prone to wound complications, dehiscence, and infections. In addition, there are always chances of persistence of nonunion/delayed union. These patients must be followed up at regular intervals and a comprehensive clinical and radiological evaluation must be obtained at every follow-up.

This patient was followed up at 6-week intervals until there were clinical and radiographical signs of healing. At 3 months, the patient had significant reduction in pain with radiographical signs of fracture healing (Fig. 20.5a, b) and at 6 months, the patient returned to full activities including running (Fig. 20.6a, b).

Pearls and Pitfalls

- Nonunion is diagnosed when no healing is noted on follow-up radiographs, provided a minimum of 6 months have passed since the initial surgery barring those with bone loss.
- All patients with nonunion should have work up for infection in the form of laboratory tests including white cell count and ESR and CRP.
- If present, infection must be appropriately treated or controlled before attempting internal fixation or bone grafting.
- Principles of surgery include stimulation of bone healing in the presence of atrophic nonunion, and achieving bony stability to allow for healing to progress.

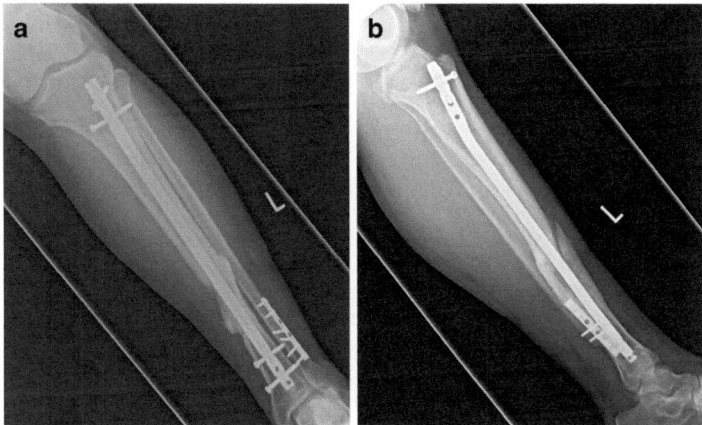

Fig. 20.5 (**a**, **b**) Three-month postoperative AP and lateral radiographic images showing good alignment, fragment contact, and evidence of healing

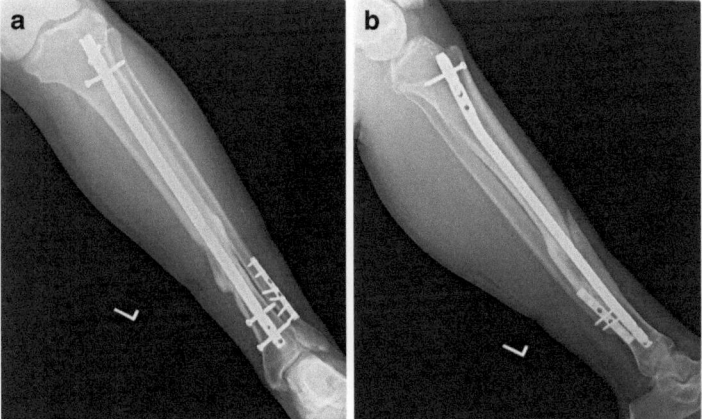

Fig. 20.6 (**a**, **b**) Six-month postoperative AP and lateral radiographic images showing fracture consolidation

References

1. Calori GM, Albisetti W, Agus A, Iori S, Tagliabue L. Risk factors contributing to fracture non-unions. Injury. 2007;38 Suppl 2:S11–8. Review. Erratum in: Injury. 2007;38(10):1224.
2. Alan K. Stotts, Peter M. Stevens. Tibial rotational osteotomy with intramedullary nail fixation. Strateg Trauma Limb Reconstr. 2009;4(3):129–33.
3. Sen M.K, Miclau T. Autologous iliac crest bone graft: should it still be the gold standard for treating nonunion? Injury. 2007;38: S75–S80.
4. Nadkarni B, Srivastav S, Mittal V, et al. Use of locking compression plates for long bone nonunions without removing existing intramedullary nail: review of literature and our experience. J Trauma. 2008;65:482–6.
5. Duan X, Al-Qwbani M, Zeng Y, Zhang W, Xiang Z. Intramedullary nailing for tibial shaft fractures in adults. Cochrane Database Syst Rev. 2012;(1):CD008241.
6. Reichert IL, McCarthy ID, Hughes SP. The acute vascular response to intramedullary reaming: microsphere estimation of blood flow in the intact bovine tibia. J Bone Joint Surg [Br]. 1995;77-B:490–3.
7. Bhandari M, Guyatt G.H, Tong D, et al. Reamed versus nonreamed intramedullary nailing of lower extremity long bone fractures: a systematic overview and meta-analysis. J Orthop Trauma. 2000;14:2–9.
8. Cannada LK, Anglen JO, Archdeacon MT, Herscovici Jr D, Ostrum RF. Avoiding complications in the care of fractures of the tibia. Instr Course Lect. 2009;58:27–36.
9. Bishop JA, Palanca AA, Bellino MJ, et al. Assessment of compromised fracture healing. J Am Acad Orthop Surg. 2012;20:273–82.
10. Hak DJ, Fitzpatrick D, Bishop JA, Marsh JL, Tilp S, Schnettler R, Simpson H, Alt V. Delayed union and nonunions: epidemiology, clinical issues, and financial aspects. Injury. 2014;45 Suppl 2:S3–7.

Chapter 21
Technique of Masquelet Bone Grafting

Philip R. Wolinksy

Case Presentation

The patient is a 28-year-old male who sustained an open right proximal tibia and fibula fracture, as a result of a motorcycle accident, which was treated with irrigation and debridement (I+D) as well as an acute open reduction internal fixation on July 13, 2007. He was transferred to the plastic surgery service at my hospital for treatment of a "chronic wound with exposed hardware," which had been treated with repeated operative debridements and placement of a wound VAC on August 24, 2007, a little over a month or so after his initial injury.

Orthopedic surgery was consulted intraoperatively by the plastic surgery service at the time of his second operative debridement for what appeared to be a necrotic bone. Cultures taken at the time of his first I+D were already growing multiple organisms. I found a large open wound on the anterior and medial aspect of the tibia that extended from just below the tibial tubercle to about two-thirds of the way down the tibia.

P.R. Wolinksy
Professor of Orthopedic Surgery,
Chief Orthopedic Trauma Service, Vice Chair Department
of Orthopedic Surgery, University of California
at Sacramento Medical Center, Sacramento, CA, USA
e-mail: philipwolinsky@hotmail.com

© Springer International Publishing Switzerland 2016   235
N.C. Tejwani (ed.), *Fractures of the Tibia: A Clinical Casebook*,
DOI 10.1007/978-3-319-21774-1_21

The exposed bone with lag screws in it did not bleed at all, and there was no granulation tissue over these areas, which made me quite suspicious that this bone was not alive (Fig. 21.1a–e). I elevated some of the granulation tissue off of the bone, and found that the fragments that had lag screws in it were obviously dead. When I used a saline-cooled burr with irrigation to look at the exposed tibia, I found that it did not bleed until I got down to the area where the wound was not open. Since the patient had a multiple-organism infection with a large soft tissue defect, I felt that he would require debridement back to healthy living tissue in an attempt to salvage his limb. The infection would likely not be able to be cured with avascular bone, soft tissue, or hardware in place. Therefore, we made a decision to proceed with aggressive I&D in an attempt to salvage his leg.

Treatment and Timing of This Surgery

The patient was already in the operating room. The goal at this point is to control the infection by removing any nonviable tissue as well as the hardware, stabilize the extremity, and treat the infection with systemic as well as local antibiotics.

Surgical Tact

Position

Supine, with a platform under the limb to elevate it above the level of the contralateral limb for imaging.

Equipment

Radiolucent table, C-arm imaging, external fixation set, hardware removal set, high-speed burr, PMMA and powdered antibiotics, irrigation solution and device, wound VAC.

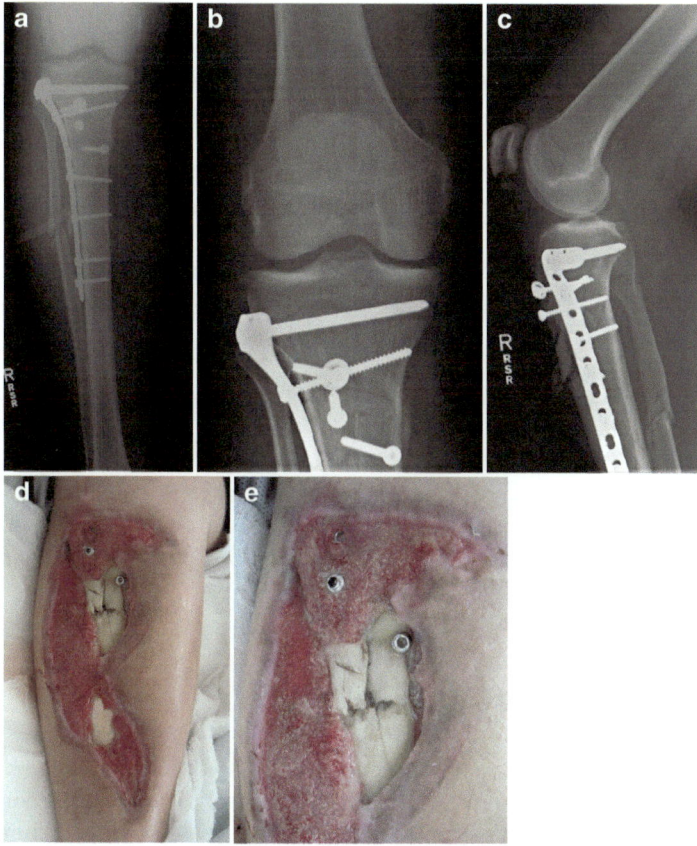

Fig. 21.1 (**a**) AP X-ray of the tibia when the patient presented to our hospital. The fracture is well reduced and is stabilized with a laterally based plate as well as three lag screws. Note that one of the lag screws is heading from medial to lateral. It was either placed percutaneously or perhaps through a large soft tissue dissection. (**b**) AP view of the knee. (**c**) Lateral view of the proximal tibia at time of presentation. (**d**) Intraoperative photograph of the wound. There is exposed bone that is not covered by any granulation tissue. There is no healing at 1 month with the fracture lines still fully visible and the bone appears desiccated. (**e**) Close-up intraoperative photo

A spanning external fixator was placed with two pins in the distal femur and two pins in the distal tibia to provide temporary stability. We then removed the hardware. Before the external fixator was placed, I stressed the leg using fluoroscopy, and found that the hardware was obviously loose and not stabilizing the fracture. The butterfly fragments were able to be taken out of the wound without any difficulty since they had no soft tissue attachments, and were avascular. A saline-cooled saw was used to cut the tibial shaft just above the point where it was avascular. This was determined by using the burr until the bone began to bleed, indicating that the blood supply was still intact.

All nonviable soft tissues were debrided as well. The wound was irrigated with copious amounts of sterile saline solution.

Antibiotic polymethylmethacrylate (PMMA) beads impregnated with tobramycin and vancomycin were placed into the bony defect, and a VAC dressing was placed over the wound. All the bone as well as the soft tissues that were left behind appeared to be grossly viable (Fig. 21.2).

Follow-Up Surgery

After surgery, the plastic surgeon and I spoke with the patient and his family about the options of amputation versus reconstruction/limb salvage, and they elected to proceed with limb salvage.

Two days later, he returned to the OR for another I + D as well as a PMMA bead exchange, and all the bony and soft tissue appeared to be viable. He returned to the OR 7 days later for soft-tissue coverage; however, some residual infection was encountered, and his wound was redebrided. Five days after that, he returned to the OR for free soft-tissue coverage with a latissimus dorsi flap as well as a split-thickness skin graft (STSG), combined with a plate fixation of the proximal tibia and placement of a PMMA antibiotic-impregnated block into the 15 cm bony defect to hold the space open for future bone grafting as well as generation of a biochemically active membrane around the periphery of the block (Figs. 21.3a, b and 21.4a–e).

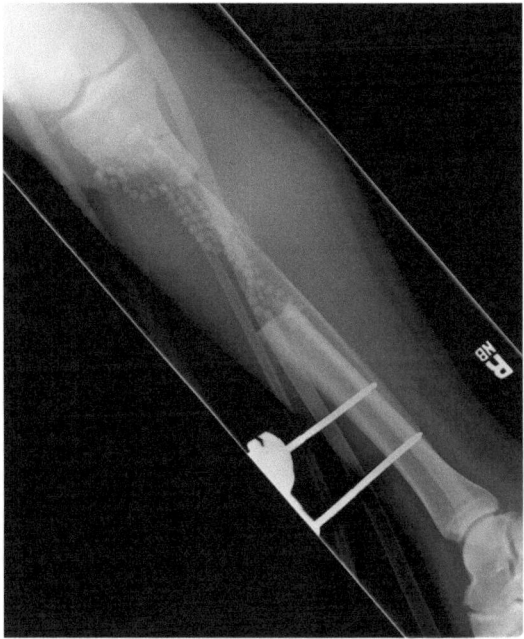

Fig. 21.2 AP X-ray of the tibia taken after the first debridement. All the hardware has been removed, an external fixator has been placed for stabilization, and antibiotic PMMA beads have been placed into the bony defect

The patient was sent home on culture-specific antibiotics. His cultures grew *E. faecalis* and MSSA, and infectious disease recommended treating him with Zosyn for 6 weeks.

Position

Supine, with a platform under the limb to elevate it above the level of the contralateral limb for imaging.

Equipment

Radiolucent table, C-arm imaging, proximal tibia locking plate set, high-speed burr, PMMA and powdered antibiotics, irrigation solution and device.

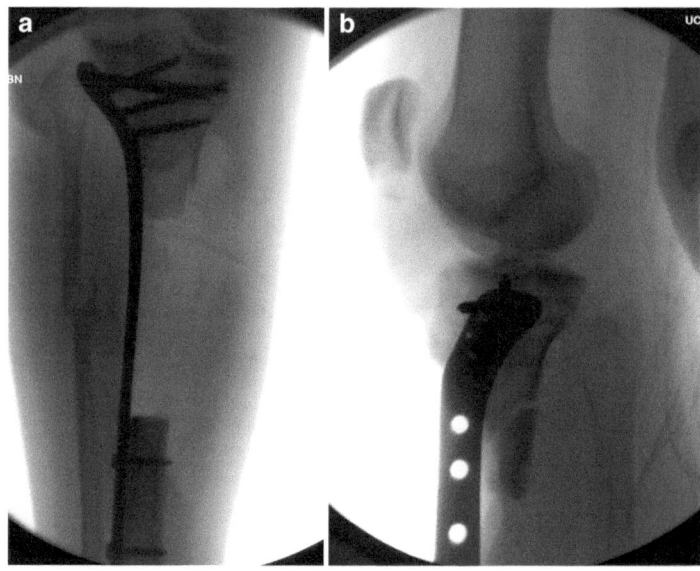

Fig. 21.3 (**a**) Intraoperative C arm AP image of the proximal tibia after resta-bilization of the fracture with a laterally based locking plate. The size of the bony defect can be appreciated. (**b**) Intraoperative lateral view

Timing

After wound healing and completion of appropriate infection treatment.

He finished his antibiotics, and his wound did not appear to be infected. ID then recommended the patient to take oral antibiotics for the remainder of his life. It took approximately 4 months (February 19, 2008) until his flap healed in to the point where it could be reelevated for bone grafting of the bony defect. X-rays at this point showed a large PMMA spacer in place with some bone attempting to bridge medially and posteriorly. At this point, the patient was scheduled for bone grafting. I talked to him about the various bone grafts available and we decided to go with allograft and BMP-2, which was my choice for massive bone grafts at the time (Fig. 21.5a, b).

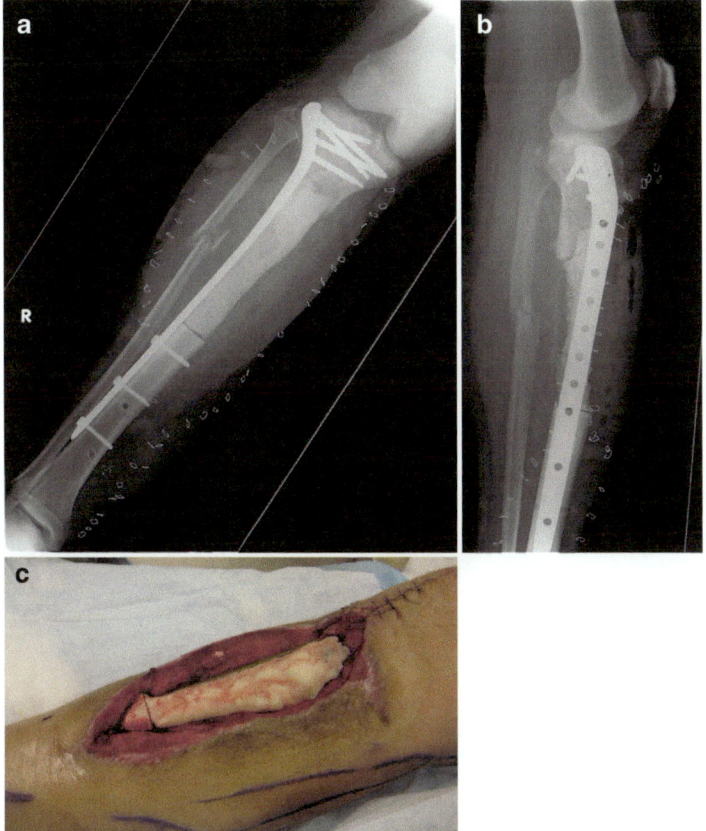

Fig. 21.4 (**a**) Post flap/re-stabilization/ insertion of PMMA bone block into the bony defect AP view of the tibia. (**b**) Lateral view of the same. (**c–e**) Intraoperative photos of the large PMMA block placed into the bony defect and the soft tissue flap

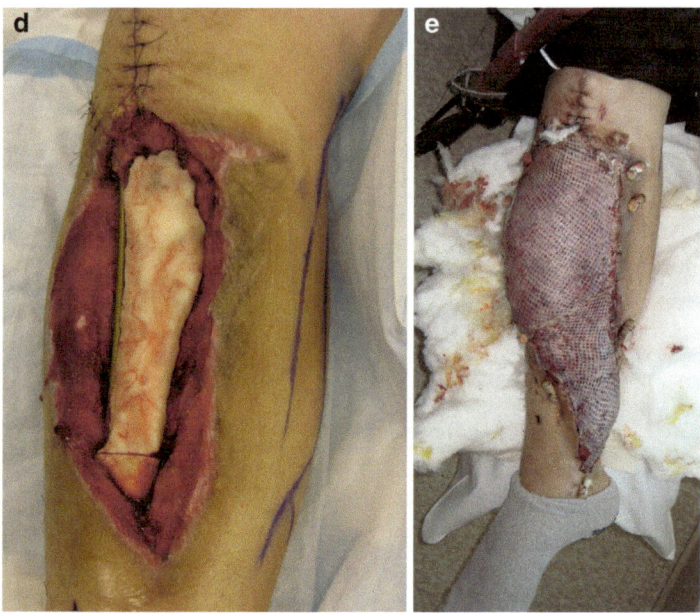

Fig. 21.4 (continued)

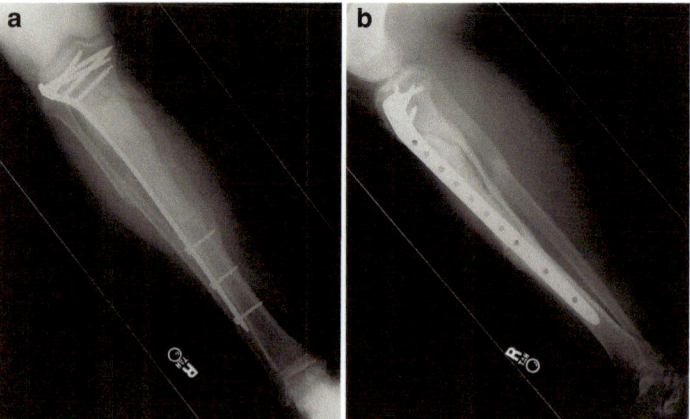

Fig. 21.5 (**a**) AP X-ray of the tibia just prior to bone grafting. There is some medial-sided bone forming. (**b**) Lateral view of the tibia showing posterior bone forming and the PMMA bone block present anterior to that bone

He was taken back to the operating room on March 21, 2008, about 5 ½ months after his soft-tissue coverage for grafting of his 15-cm bone deficit. The flap was raised along its anterolateral border, going directly down to bone and cement, raising the flap as a single unit without tension. The antibiotic spacer was exposed and removed. The proximal and distal ends of the bone were scraped with a curette to remove any intervening fibrous tissue, and the distal end of the canal was then drilled with a cooled drill bit until good bleeding was seen. Deep cultures were sent.

Fluoroscopy was used to make sure that all the cement had been removed. We then began grafting with cancellous allograft. There was a nice shell of fibrous tissue and bone into which the graft was to be placed. The bone graft was impacted using a bone tamp, and we used fluoroscopy to insure that the entire defect was filled.

We then laid a BMP2-impregnated sponge over the visible area of the allograft (Fig. 21.6a, b). His cultures ended up being negative, and he was discharged on his oral antibiotics.

When he was seen at 2 months following surgery, he was made partial weight-bearing; at 3 months (June 17, 2008), he was made weight-bearing as tolerated. At 5 months (September 11, 2008), he had some interval filling-in of his bone graft and reported that he felt he was doing quite well. He had some swelling in his leg, had regained a lot of his mobility, but was still having issues with strength.

At about 10 months after grafting (February 5, 2009), he was back working as a security guard for up to 10 h a day or more. He reported that after 10 h or so of being up on his leg, his leg starts hurting. He had been seen by Infectious Disease recently who felt there was no evidence of infection, and they discontinued his antibiotics A sedimentation rate (ESR) and C-reactive protein (CRP) were normal and unchanged from his prior values. He has no history of fevers or of drainage.

On physical exam, there was no erythema, drainage, or other signs suggestive of infection. His X-rays showed no loosening or halo effect around his screws or any loss of reduction. On the lateral view, there was a posterior shelf of bone. At this point, I thought the patient was doing well considering the size of the defect that he had and that he was still healing and remodeling. He had no ability to modify his job to work less hours per day or at a less physically demanding job.

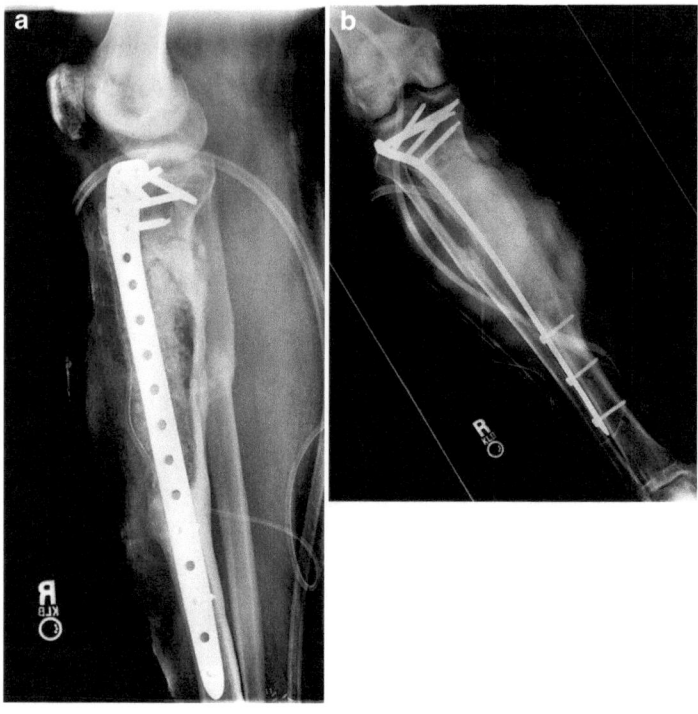

Fig. 21.6 (**a**) Lateral view of the tibia just after removal of the PMMA bone block and bone grafting with cancellous allograft. The posterior cortex bony bridge can be seen. (**b**) AP X-ray of the tibia just after bone grafting of the defect

He was next seen about 1 year out from surgery (March 2, 2010). The patient felt he was doing well, was now working as a wine bottler and was able to be up on his feet for 8–12 h a day. His soft tissues were intact with no erythema, no drainage, or other signs of infection, and his X-rays showed further remodeling of his bone graft (Fig. 21.7a, b).

About 3 months later (June 15, 2010), he developed pain and erythema of his leg and was admitted for an I + D. A CT scan did not reveal a fluid collection. He was started on empiric IV antibiotics, improved dramatically and was discharged without needing surgery on antibiotics for 6 weeks (Figs. 21.8a, b and 21.9a, b).

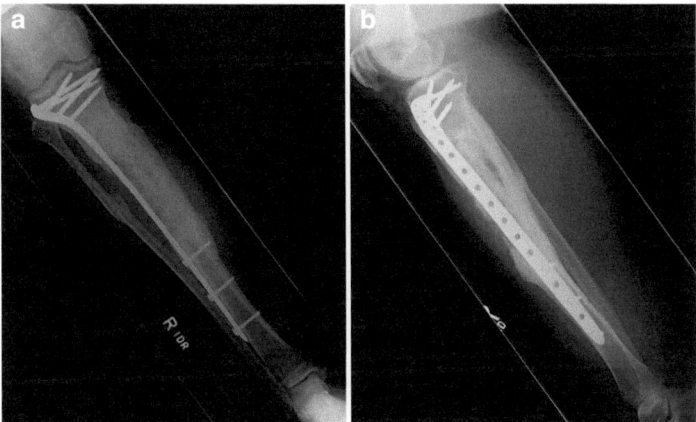

Fig. 21.7 (**a**) AP view of the tibia 12 months after bone grafting showing what appears to be incorporation of the graft. (**b**) Lateral view of the tibia at the same time showing hypertrophy of the posterior cortex and graft incorporation

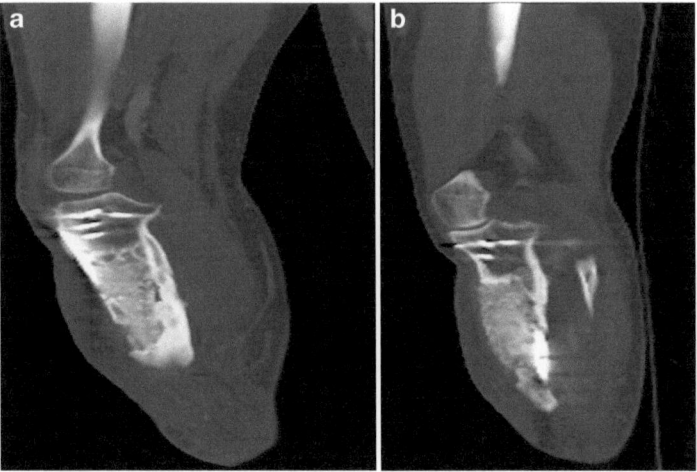

Fig. 21.8 (**a**) Lateral reconstruction CT view showing how much of the graft is actually not incorporated. (**b**) AP CT reconstruction showing the same

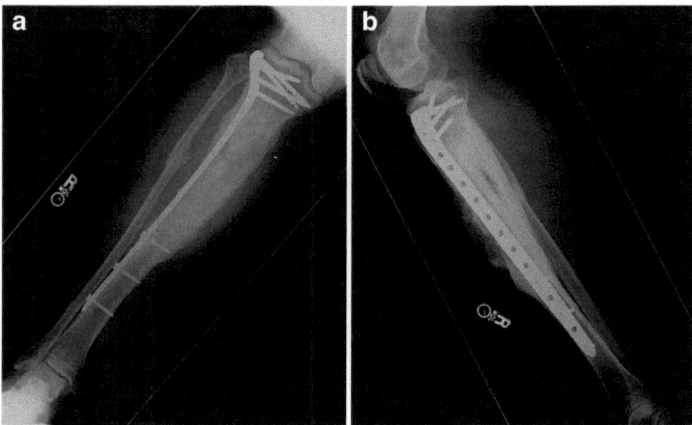

Fig. 21.9 (**a**) AP view of the tibia at 20 months after grafting just prior to I + D. (**b**) Lateral view at the same time

However, he subsequently developed a draining sinus and was brought to the operating room for an I + D, exploration, removal of hardware, and placement of antibiotic-impregnated beads on November 10, 2010. At the time of surgery, he had some gross purulence as well as some loose unincorporated bone graft that were removed, but his posterior and anterior cortices were healed. He was not healed laterally or medially. There was about a 10-cm central defect (Fig. 21.10a–e). The limb was grossly stable on physical exam, as well as on fluoroscopic exam. We therefore elected not to stabilize it at this point in the setting of an active infection. His cultures were negative, but, since he had been on antibiotics prior to surgery, they were empirically continued post-operatively for 6 weeks.

My intention was to go back and regraft him; however, the patient felt so well after surgery that he was able to be up on his feet, working 10–12 h a day, and he never would let me do it. I last saw him on November 13, 2014 – almost 6 years after his bone grafting. He was working full time as a bottling plant engineer, which requires him to be on his feet and kneeling for long periods of time. Imaging revealed hypertrophy of the healed cortexes (Fig. 21.11a, b).

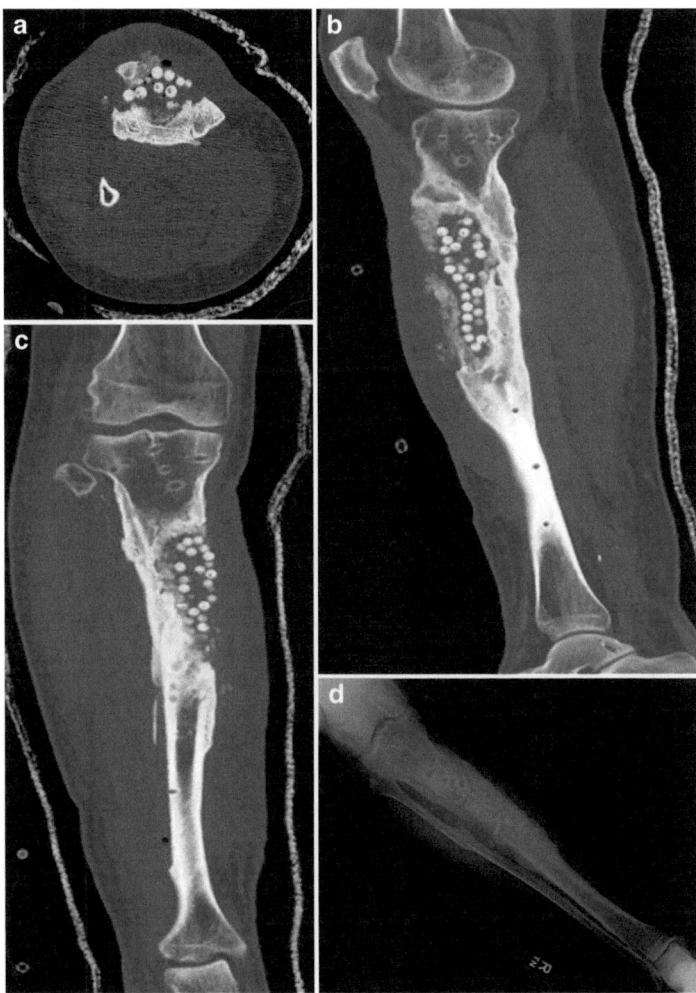

Fig. 21.10 (**a**) Axial CT cut after I+D showing the extent of the intact posterior cortex. (**b**) Lateral CT reconstruction. (**c**) AP CT reconstruction showing
the lateral cortex. (**d**) Compare the CT to the AP plain film view. (**e**) And the
lateral plain film view

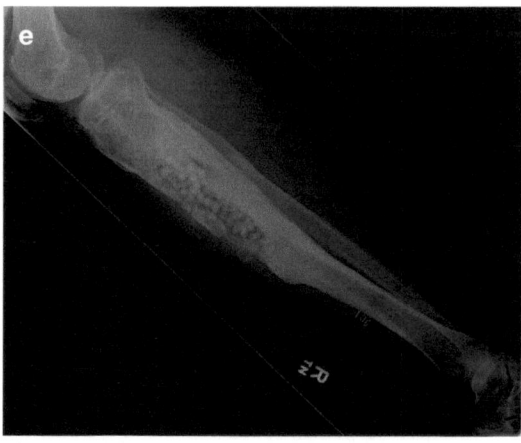

Fig. 21.10 (continued)

Introduction/Summary/Salient Tips/Pearls

- This case is an illustration of the Masquelet technique for bone grafting.
- The concept is to create a membrane-encased space for bone grafting. The membrane that surrounds the defect is thought to be biochemically active and to create an environment that is conducive and hospitable for incorporation of bone graft. The original series described using autograft for the bone graft.
- I have evolved in what graft I prefer to use. At the time that I took care of this patient, I was using pure allograft with bone-morphogenic protein (BMP-2).
- Currently, I tend to use autograft obtained using the RIA (reamer irrigator aspirator) technique and use allograft as a graft expanded is needed based on the size of the defect. In addition, I used a plate for this patient, but now prefers to use an intramedullary nail if possible since the central part of the graft may not be as well vascularized as the periphery and tends not to incorporate as well as the graft distributed around the periphery. For the same reason, I do not pack the graft in as tightly as I used to in the past, hoping that it will allow for greater revascularization of the graft.

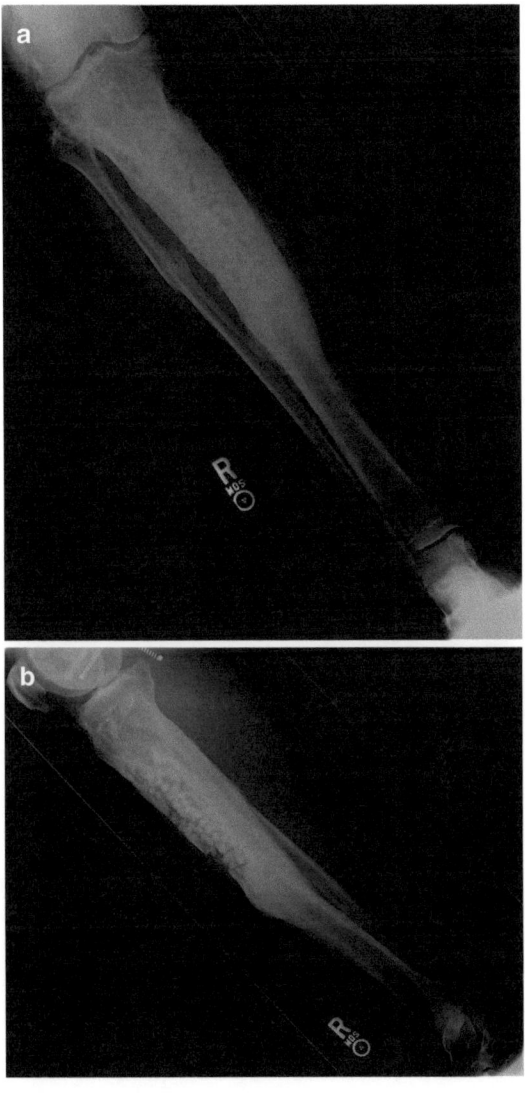

Fig. 21.11 (**a**) AP view of the tibia 6 years after bone grafting with thick medial and lateral cortexes. (**b**) Lateral view showing the impressive hypertrophy of the posterior cortex

Bibliography

1. Christou C, Oliver RA, Yu Y, Walsh WR. The masquelet technique for membrane induction and the healing of ovine critical sized segmental defects. PLoS One. 2014;9(12):e114122.
2. Gouron R, Petit L, Boudot C, Six I, Brazier M, Kamel S, Mentaverri R. Osteoclasts and their precursors are present in the induced-membrane during bone reconstruction using the Masquelet technique. J Tissue Eng Regen Med. 2014. Article first published online: 12 JUN 2014. DOI:10.1002/term.1921.
3. Aho O, Lehenkari P, Ristiniemi J, Lehtonen S, Risteli J, Leskelä H. The mechanism of action of induced membranes in bone repair. J Bone Joint Surg Am. 2013;95(7):597–604.
4. Giannoudis PV, Faour O, Goff T, Kanakaris K, Dimitriou R. Masquelet technique for the treatment of bone defects: tips-tricks and future directions. Injury. 2011;42(6):591–8.

Chapter 22
Modified Clamshell Osteotomy for Treating Acute Tibial Shaft Fracture with Pre-existent Malunion

Namdar Kazemi, Rafael Kakazu, and Michael T. Archdeacon

Case Presentation

The patient is a 56-year-old female with a history of schizoaffective disorder and multiple medical comorbidities who presented complaining of leg pain attributed to a fall while getting out of bed.

Injury Films

Radiographs demonstrated a spiral distal tibial shaft fracture, as well as a segmental right fibular fracture. Surgical treatment with an intramedullary nail was recommended because of concern for noncompliance with closed treatment. The patient refused surgical intervention citing fear of complications. She was treated in a closed manner with a long-leg cast with acceptable alignment

N. Kazemi, MD • R. Kakazu, MD (✉)
M.T. Archdeacon, MD, MSE
Department of Orthopaedic Surgery, University of Cincinnati
College of Medicine, 231 Albert Sabin Way ML 0212,
Cincinnati, OH 45267-0212, USA
e-mail: Rafael.Kakazu@UC.edu

© Springer International Publishing Switzerland 2016   251
N.C. Tejwani (ed.), *Fractures of the Tibia: A Clinical Casebook*,
DOI 10.1007/978-3-319-21774-1_22

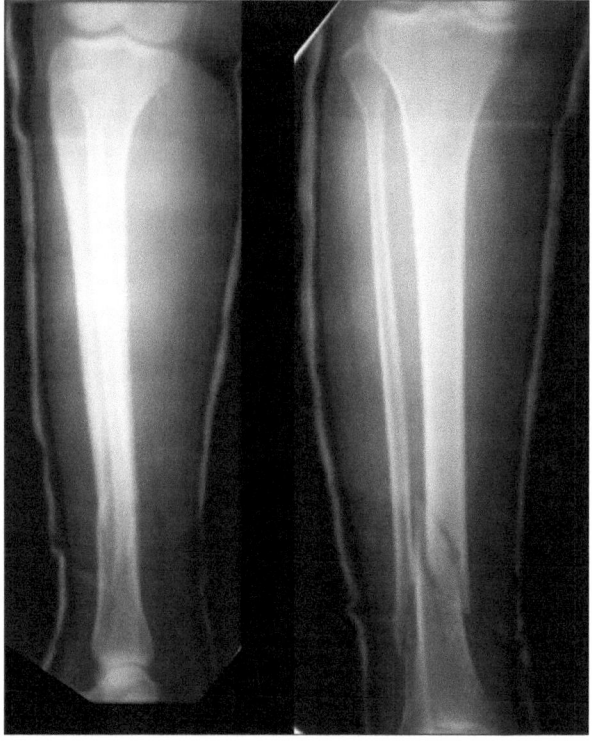

Fig. 22.1 AP and lateral radiographs demonstrating a spiral distal tibial shaft fracture and segmental right fibular fracture. The patient was treated in a closed manner with a long-leg cast with acceptable alignment

(Fig. 22.1). Radiographs obtained at 6-month follow-up exhibited extensive callus formation with moderate malalignment including 25 % lateral displacement and approximately 15° of recurvatum (Fig. 22.2).

Seven months after the initial fracture, the patient presented to the emergency department with new onset pain after a fall. Radiographs demonstrated an acute oblique tibia fracture proximal to the prior tibial malunion. An associated acute spiral fracture of the fibula was noted (Fig. 22.3).

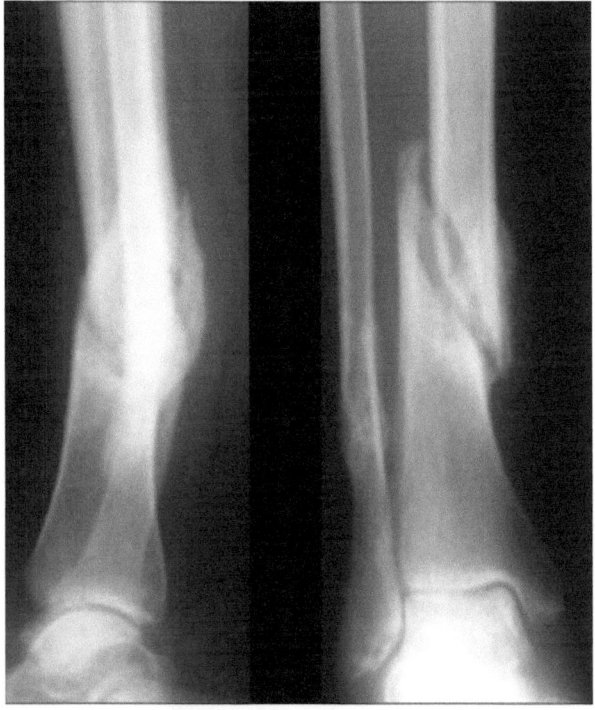

Fig. 22.2 At 6 months following the injury, AP and lateral radiographs exhibited extensive callus formation with moderate malalignment including 22 % lateral displacement and approximately 15° of recurvatum

Treatment Considerations/Planning/Tests Needed

Treatment options were discussed, and the patient decided to proceed with operative treatment. In order to realign the tibia and obtain stable fixation of the acute fracture, a modified Russell "clam-shell" osteotomy with intramedullary fixation of the tibia was considered.

One of the challenges in this scenario is that the preexisting deformity essentially distorts the intramedullary canal, precluding the passage of an intramedullary nail. Traditional treatment options such as wedge osteotomy, dome osteotomy, and distraction

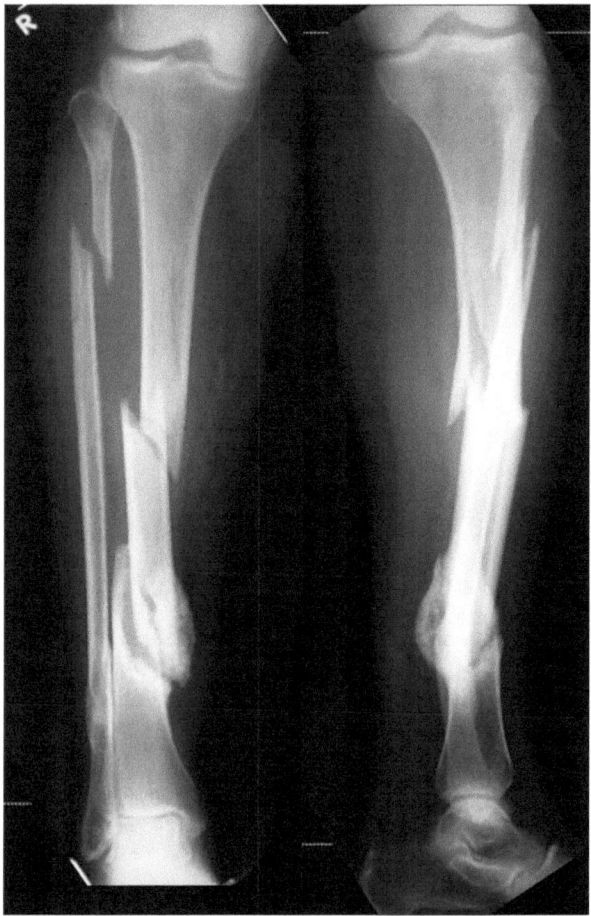

Fig. 22.3 AP and lateral radiographs demonstrating an acute oblique tibia shaft fracture proximal to the previous tibial malunion. An associated acute spiral fracture of the fibula was noted

osteogenesis are complex, technically demanding, and associated with complications [1–4]. In an effort to simplify deformity correction, a modified Russell clamshell osteotomy [5] with intramedullary nail stabilization is proposed. The procedure is modified in the sense that instead of performing both a proximal and distal osteotomy, the acute fracture is utilized as the proximal osteotomy limb and a single distal osteotomy is performed. The clamshell segment effectively bypasses the malunion by realigning the mechanical axis of the extremity. The intramedullary nail maintains length, alignment, and rotation while allowing early weight bearing.

Contraindications to this technique include a poor soft tissue envelope and extensive bone shortening due to the malunion. The muscular envelope around the tibia is limited and soft tissue integrity plays an important role for the surgical approach to the malunion site. The surgeon should be aware of and plan for the possible need for soft tissue coverage after deformity correction. Correction of deformities with extensive shortening poses a risk to the neurovascular structures and should be avoided. Russell et al. recommended no more than 3 cm of length correction of the tibia in their original study [5].

Preoperative evaluation provides information about the malunion and the acute fracture for an improved understanding for the deformity. Lower limb discrepancy can be determined by comparing the measured distance between the anterior superior iliac spine to the tip of the medial malleolus of each extremity. If the limblength inequality is greater than 2.5 cm, a scanogram is recommended. Particular attention should be paid to the soft tissue zone over the segment of the deformity as well as the acute fracture. Rotational profile is determined with the extremity in the supine resting position. The thigh-foot axis is used to assess tibial torsion. Radiographs are used to evaluate the character of the malunion and the proximal and distal joints. Coronal and sagittal angulation can be determined by the angle formed by the intersection of the anatomic axes of the proximal and distal segments. Translation along the coronal and sagittal plane is calculated from the perpendicular distance between the anatomic axis of the proximal segment and the anatomic axis of the distal segment when translational and angular deformities are present.

Timing of Surgery

Given the fact that the patient had a psychiatric disorder and a concern that the patient may not return for follow-up, operative stabilization was deemed the safest option. Additionally, the patient preferred operative treatment to nonoperative treatment. Discussed in detail with the patient was the need for compliance with a nonoperative treatment regimen including routine interval follow-up for cast care and radiographs. Once operative treatment is chosen, the timing for surgical intervention is dependent on the soft tissue envelope and medical optimization. This is particularly relevant in a patient who is a poor patient historian and who has multiple medical comorbidities. With no evidence of neurovascular injury, no evidence of an impending compartment syndrome, and minimal soft tissue edema to the limb and optimization of medical problems, surgery was performed within 24 h of injury.

Intraoperative Tips and Tricks for Reduction/ Fixation

Position

Supine with radiolucent bump for flexing the knee to allow tibial nailing.

Approach

A standard tibial intramedullary nailing was initiated through a medial parapatellar entrance. After a guide wire was placed into the proximal tibia, reaming was initiated in the proximal segment up to the level of the fracture.

Fracture Reduction

A 2-cm anteromedial incision at the level of the acute fracture was made with subperiosteal exposure of the tibial shaft. Next, the distal portion of the malunion was exposed subperiosteally through a separate incision. A transverse osteotomy of the tibia was performed just distal to the malunion, oriented parallel to the ankle joint (Fig. 22.4a–c). The intercalary segment between the acute fracture and the distal tibial transverse osteotomy was serially drilled along the anteromedial cortex with a 3.5 mm drill-bit, and subsequently split longitudinally in the anteromedial plane using an osteotome (Fig. 22.4d, e). The anterior cortex of the intercalary segment was separated with a lamina spreader and the posterior cortex hinged on the periosteum; thus, the "clamshell" osteotomy as described by Russell et al. [5] (Fig. 22.4f). The ball-tip guide wire was passed through the osteotomized intercalary segment and into the distal tibia. Care was taken to ensure that the guide wire was centered in the distal tibial metaphysis in both AP and lateral views [4]. Reaming was then continued, starting with a 9 mm reamer, advancing in half-millimeter increments up to 12 mm. The clamshell segment was not reamed; rather, the reamer was pushed through the clamshell segment to avoid injury to surrounding neurovascular structures. Successive reamings will usually produce sufficient bone fragments to fill the osteotomy sites. After good cortical chatter was appreciated, an appropriately sized intramedullary nail was inserted over the guide wire, through the osteotomized segment and into the distal tibia (Fig. 22.4g). Then, static locking screws were placed both proximally and distally (Fig. 22.5a, b). Before closing, the osteotomy sites should be inspected for gaps. If there is a gap of more than 1 cm, autogenous bone graft should be considered to ensure no space between the osteotomy fragments and the intact proximal or distal parts of the tibia. The fascia should be approximated loosely. If there is concern for excessive swelling that may contribute to compartment syndrome, the anterior compartment fascia should not be closed. We recommend closure of the incision using the Allgower modification of the Donati technique, with particular emphasis on careful soft tissue handling. Once the incision is closed, a sterile compressive dressing and a well-padded posterior splint were applied.

Postoperative Plan

The patient should be closely monitored for sign and symptoms of compartment syndrome. Regional block anesthesia is denied for more effective evaluation. Concern for compartment syndrome must be balanced with appropriate pain control. However, a high degree of suspicion for compartment syndrome and a low threshold

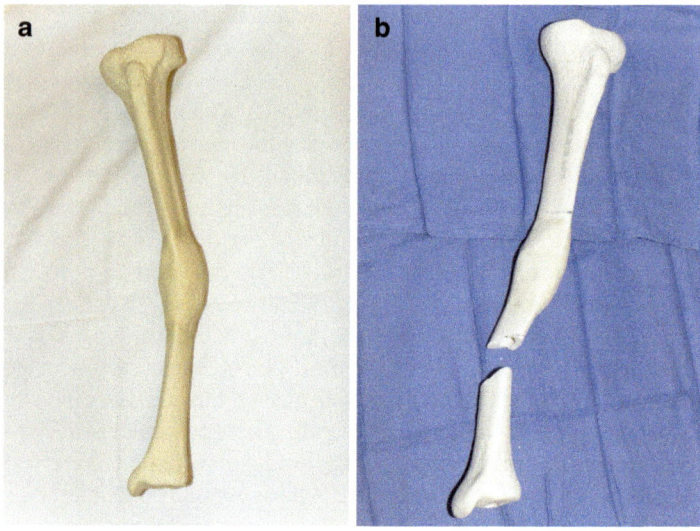

Fig. 22.4 In order to better illustrate the technique, the authors performed the procedure on a sawbones model. (**a**) A sawbones model of a left tibia with a 30° varus deformity secondary to malunion will be used to demonstrate the described technique.(**b**) A fracture is made distal to the malunion. Note the *dashed line* proximal to the malunion indicating the osteotomy site. (**c**) The transverse osteotomy has been completed. The *dotted line* running longitudinally along the intercalary segment indicates the sites for serial drilling in preparation for subsequent osteotomy. (**d**) Serial drilling of the intercalary segment has been completed. (**e**) Use of an osteotome to split the intercalary segment longitudinally in the anteromedial plane. (**f**) Use of a lamina spreader to separate the anterior cortex of the intercalary segment, completing the "clamshell" osteotomy. (**g**) Following insertion of an intramedullary nail, the initial deformity has been corrected and the fracture stabilized

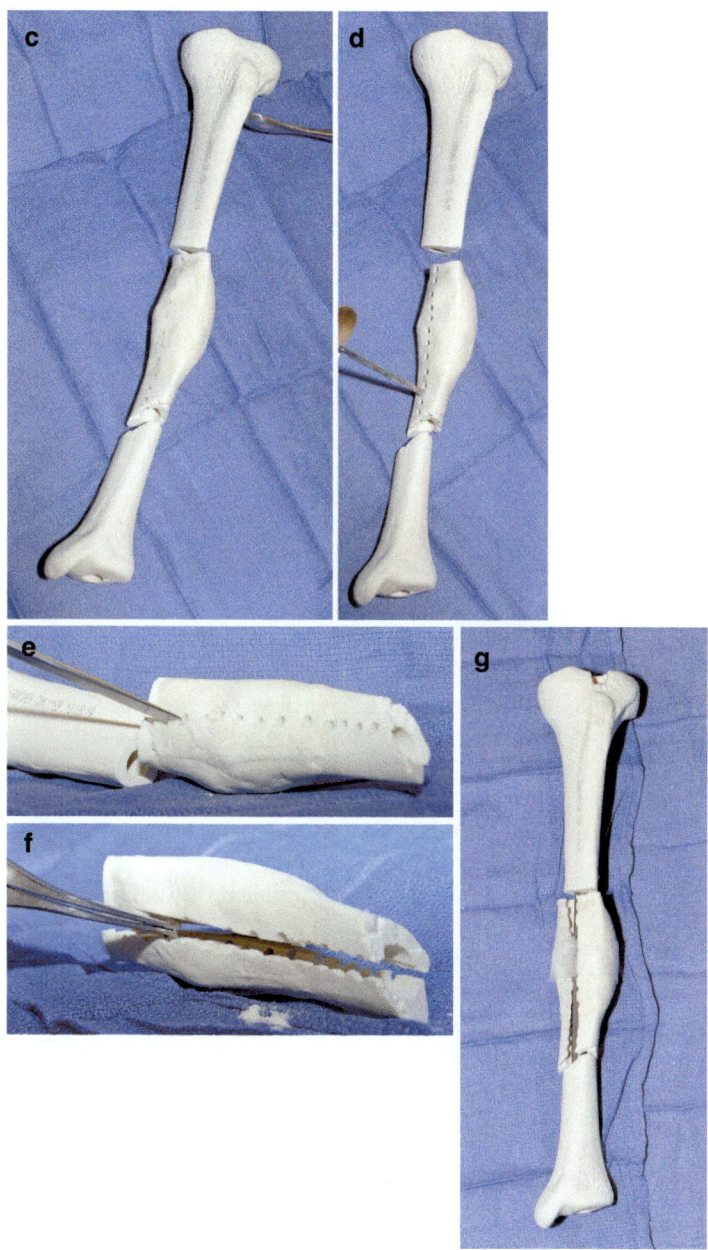

Fig. 22.4 (continued)

for fasciotomy are strongly recommended. Intravenous cefazolin is administered for three postoperative doses. On the first postoperative day, the patient is mobilized with crutches with toe-touch weight bearing. Until discharge, prophylaxis against venous thrombosis is provided by low molecular weight heparin.

Radiographs and clinical exams were performed at 7–10 days after surgery and at 4-week intervals until healing was confirmed. Physical therapy was initiated based on patient needs and was not standardized. Patient was allowed partial weight bearing until callus formation was noted on radiographs, at which time weight bearing was advanced as tolerated with a goal of full weight bearing at 12 weeks. After healing, orthogonal radiographs and standing hip-to-ankle radiographs are used to evaluate the lower extremity mechanical axis with respect to the uninjured side.

Outcome

At final follow-up, 13 months postoperative, the patient was full weight bearing with minimal complaints of pain. Biplanar radiographs demonstrated complete union of both the acute fracture and the clamshell osteotomy. The intramedullary nail was intact with acceptable translational, angular, and rotational alignment (Fig. 22.5a–d).

Salient Points/Pearls

- A unique approach to a difficult problem of fracture around a long bone malunion.
- The clamshell segment effectively bypasses the malunion by realigning the mechanical axis of the extremity.
- Contraindications to this technique include a poor soft tissue envelope and extensive bone shortening due to the malunion.
- Use of an intramedullary nail maintains length, alignment, and rotation while allowing early weight bearing as compared to open plating.
- Close follow-up is necessary to identify compartment syndrome early and delayed healing later.

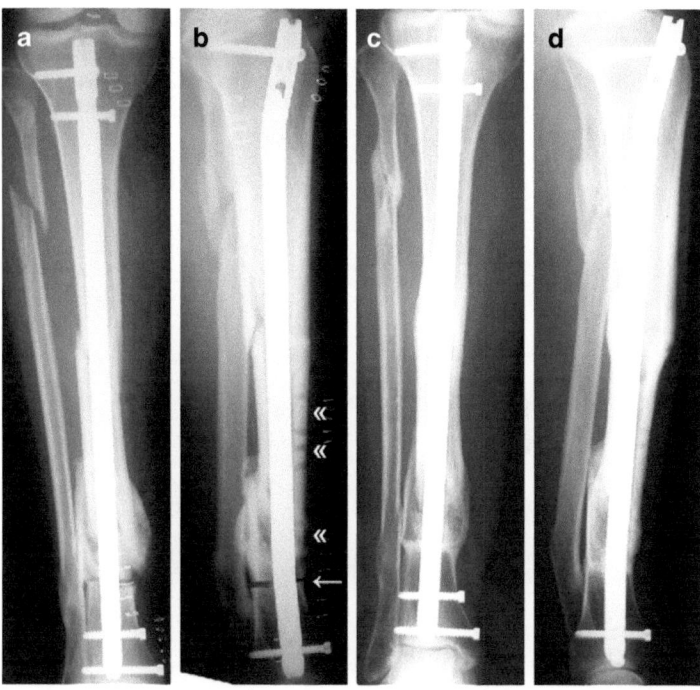

Fig. 22.5 (**a**, **b**) AP and lateral radiographs demonstrating fracture fixation with intramedullary nail. Note the distal osteotomy limb (*arrow*) and the path for the longitudinal osteotomy demarcated with a 3.5 mm drill-bit (*double arrow-heads*; «); (**c**, **d**) radiographs at final follow-up showing minimal translational, angular, and rotational deformity of the tibia

References

1. Dahl MT, Gulli B, Berg T. Complications of limb lengthening. A learning curve. Clin Orthop Relat Res. 1994;301:10–8.
2. Tetsworth K, Paley D. Malalignment and degenerative arthropathy. Orthop Clin North Am. 1994;25(3):367–77.
3. Graehl PM, Hersh MR, Heckman JD. Supramalleolar osteotomy for the treatment of symptomatic tibial malunion. J Orthop Trauma. 1987;1(4):281–92.
4. Freedman EL, Johnson EE. Radiographic analysis of tibial fracture malalignment following intramedullary nailing. Clin Orthop Relat Res. 1995;315:25–33.

5. Russell GV, Graves ML, Archdeacon MT, Barei DP, Brien GA, Porter SE. The clamshell osteotomy: a new technique to correct complex diaphyseal malunions. J Bone Joint Surg Am. 2009;91(2):314–24. doi:10.2106/JBJS.H.00158.

Chapter 23
Treatment of Tibia Malunion with Circular External Fixation

Toni M. McLaurin

Clinical History

A 33-year-old man presents with the complaint of a long-standing right ankle deformity. He had sustained an injury to his right ankle at the age of 11 or 12 when he fell off a jungle gym and "landed hard" on his right leg. At that time, he did not seek any medical care, as the assumption was that it was just an ankle sprain. Around the age of 16, he began noticing increasing deformity of his right ankle and worsening pronation in his gait. He reports being diagnosed at that time with a missed physeal injury that had resulted in a distal tibial deformity. However, he tolerated this deformity for over 15 years until he recently began noticing increasing problems with his gait including balance difficulties sometimes resulting in falls, especially while descending stairs. He also noted an occasional sensation of his ankle giving way. He presented with the question of whether or not anything could be done for this long-standing but worsening problem. His past medical history was

T.M. McLaurin, MD
Department of Orthopaedics, NYU Hospital for Joint Diseases,
550 First Avenue, BHC CD4-106, New York, NY 10016, USA
e-mail: toni.mclaurin@nyumc.org

© Springer International Publishing Switzerland 2016   263
N.C. Tejwani (ed.), *Fractures of the Tibia: A Clinical Casebook*,
DOI 10.1007/978-3-319-21774-1_23

significant only for previous tobacco use as well as previous heroin use, although he was now in recovery and gainfully employed.

On physical examination he had an obvious right ankle deformity (Fig. 23.1) with prominence of his medial distal tibia and apparent hindfoot valgus that was not correctable. He had large callosities over the medial aspect of his first metatarsal head and great toe and ambulated on the medial border of his foot with his foot pronated. Radiographs showed an 18-degree valgus deformity of the distal tibia at the level of the physeal scar consistent with a prior physeal injury (Fig. 23.2). There was no significant sagittal plane deformity and the ankle mortise was intact.

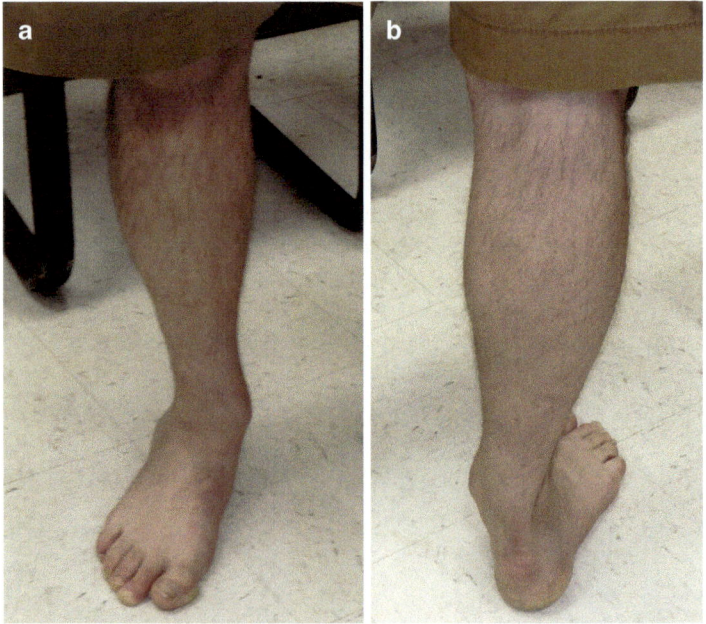

Fig. 23.1 Clinical photograph of ankle deformity as viewed from the front (**a**) and the back (**b**)

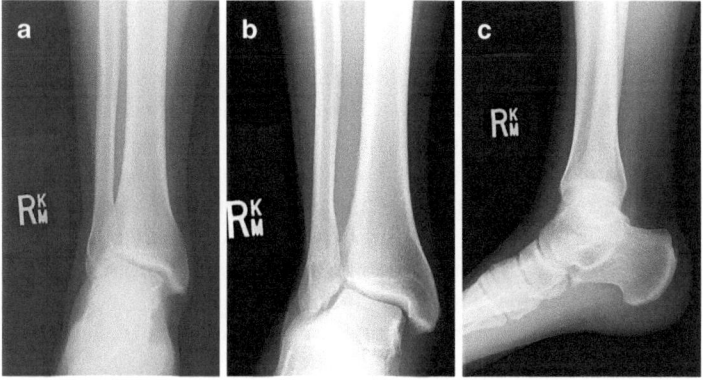

Fig. 23.2 AP (**a**), oblique (**b**) and lateral (**c**) radiographs of distal tibial physeal malunion

Treatment Considerations

The treatment options discussed with the patient included a medial closing wedge osteotomy, a lateral opening wedge osteotomy, or computer-assisted gradual correction using a circular ring external fixator (Taylor Spatial Frame, Smith and Nephew, Memphis, TN). The closing wedge osteotomy would result in a limb length discrepancy and the amount of correction would be fixed at the time of surgery and unchangeable. Similarly, the opening wedge osteotomy would result in a fixed and unchangeable initial correction and both may not adequately take into account any rotational deformity that could be present but not easily detected clinically. In addition, either option would require a prolonged period of non-weight bearing while the osteotomy healed. In contrast, the circular frame would allow a gradual correction that could be modified throughout the course of the correction to account for any deformities, such as rotation that may have initially been missed due to the more obvious valgus deformity. It would also allow full weight bearing immediately postoperatively. The obvious concern about a circular frame requiring significant patient involvement was this patient's history of heroin abuse, but he was actively in treatment for it, provided the name of his treating physician and was honest about his past relapse history. He did commit to participating fully in his care.

The only additional studies that were thought to be required preoperatively in this case were full-length tibia radiographs (Fig. 23.3), in addition to the already obtained AP, lateral, and mortise views of the ankle. Since this was not a congenital deformity and was focused about the ankle joint, there was little concern about any issues more proximally that could affect the overall limb alignment. In more complex deformities, entire leg films should be obtained and, in addition, a CT scan and especially 3-D reconstructions may be helpful to further delineate the deformity.

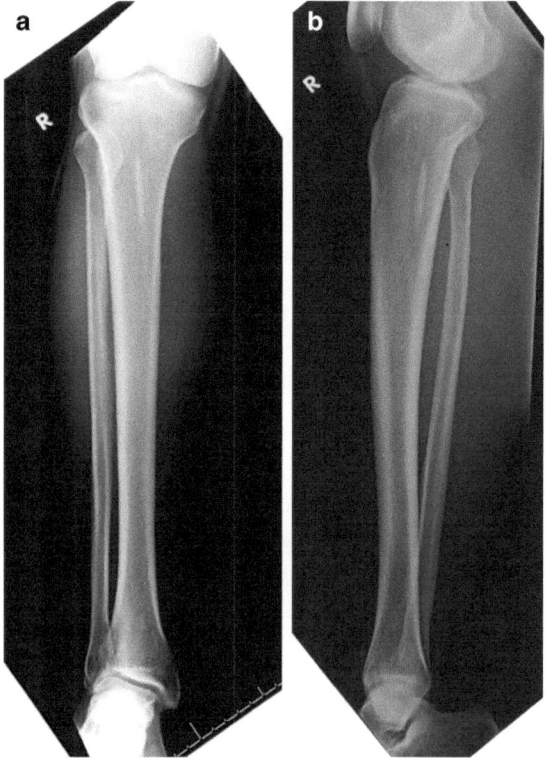

Fig. 23.3 AP (**a**) and lateral (**b**) full length tibia films to assess overall tibial alignment

Once the deformity was adequately evaluated both clinically and radiographically, the plan was made to perform a supramalleolar corticotomy, and the deformity parameters were entered into the software to appropriately prepare for the frame application and later entering of the frame mounting parameters (Fig. 23.4).

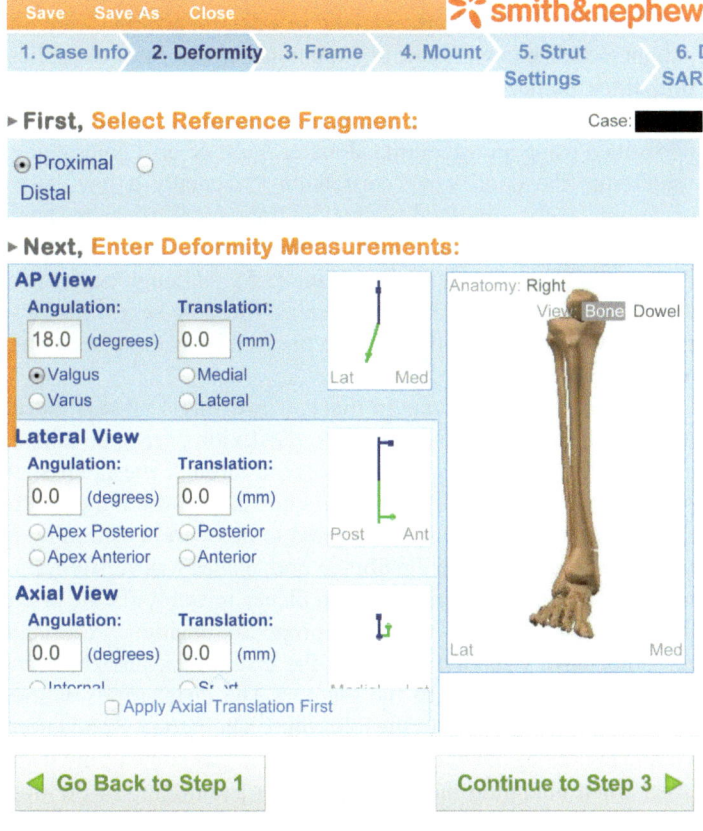

Fig. 23.4 Deformity parameters entered into computer program (Reproduced with permission: Smith and Nephew, Memphis, TN)

Timing of Surgery

There were no clinical timing issues for this chronic deformity, so timing was based on the patient's wishes.

Intraoperative Tips and Tricks

Rigorous preoperative templating and planning are essential for any deformity case. Once in the operating room, care must be taken to be sure the leg can be maintained in a neutral position while the patient is supine to eliminate any rotational errors. Prior to application of the frame, a Gigli saw was passed around the distal tibia to be used later to perform the corticotomy. Although this can also be performed using an osteotome alone or multiple drill holes and an osteotome, the Gigli saw "corticotomy" (actually a low-energy osteotomy as the endosteal tissues *are* transected) has been shown to result in decreased healing time of the regenerate bone [1, 2] and is the author's preferred method (Fig. 23.5). Although performing the corticotomy is one of the final steps, it can be very difficult to pass the Gigli saw once the frame is on, so it is always placed prior to starting the frame application.

Once the Gigli saw was in place, a two ring TSF was placed utilizing the "rings first" method. A transfixion wire to be utilized as the first "reference wire" was placed through the tibial shaft proximal to the deformity and perpendicular to the long axis of the tibia and a ring was then attached to this wire. Positioning of the ring perpendicular to the tibia in both planes was verified fluoroscopically and a half pin was then placed to stably fix the proximal ring to the tibia in the appropriate position. A second reference wire was then placed in the distal tibia, just above the ankle joint and parallel to the plafond. The distal ring was then positioned to be parallel to the joint line on both the AP and lateral views (Fig. 23.6). Due to the significant valgus slope of the distal tibia, when obtaining the lateral view for positioning of the ring, it was important to insure that the x-ray beam was aligned along the axis of the joint, and not just positioned for a standard lateral projection of the ankle to avoid malpositioning of the ring

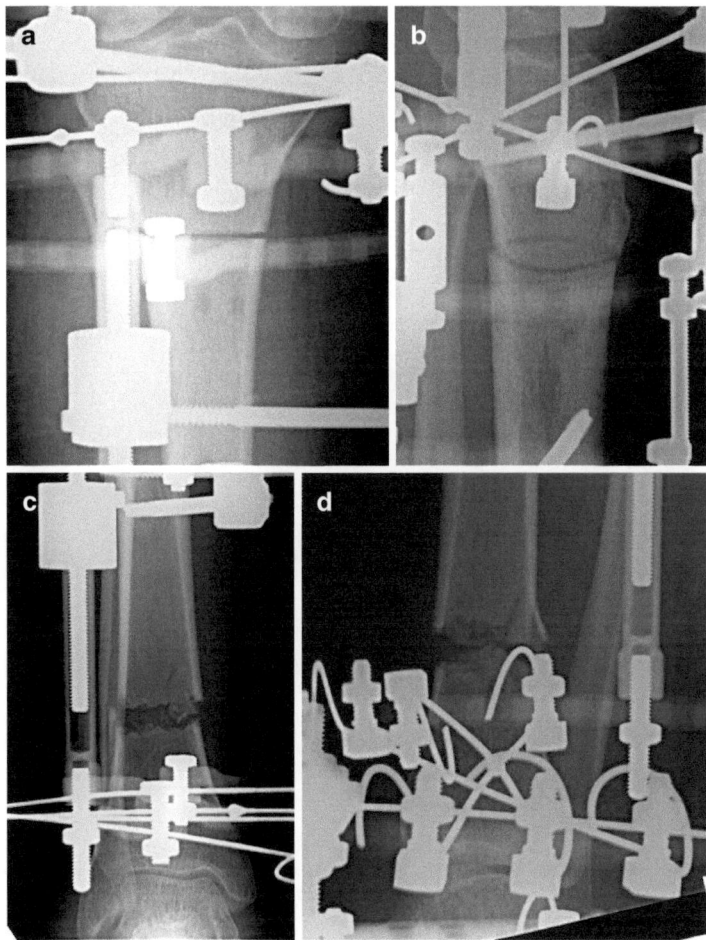

Fig. 23.5 Radiographic appearance of corticotomy made using a Gigli saw (**a**, **b**) compared to that performed with multiple drill holes and an osteotome (**c**, **d**)

(Fig. 23.7). Once appropriate positioning of this ring was confirmed, additional transfixion wires were then placed to complete the distal fixation, as metaphyseal bone does not support half pins well long-term. Two additional half pins were added to

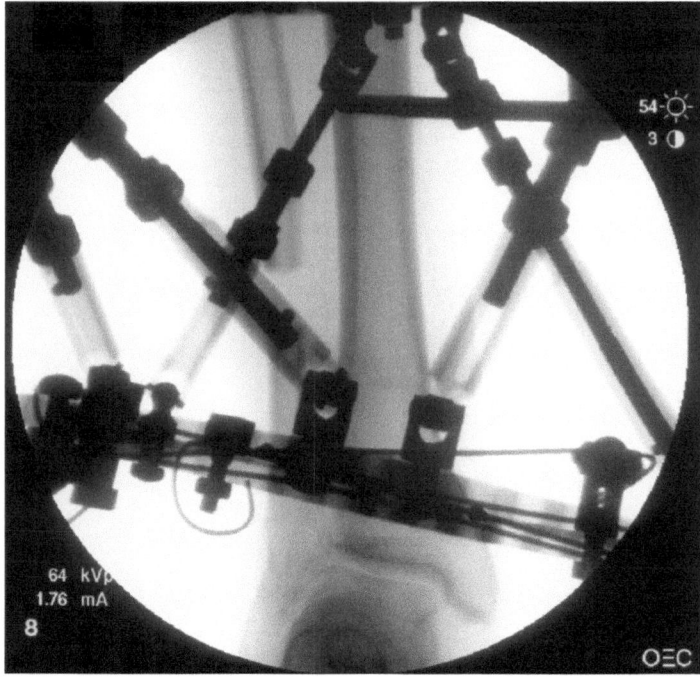

Fig. 23.6 Intra-operative fluoroscopic views of distal ring placement for the deformity. Note on the AP that the position of the frame parallels the tibial plafond

the proximal ring, and the more proximal tibial transfixion wire that had been used as a reference wire to ensure perpendicular placement of the first ring was removed, as this region of the leg does not tolerate transfixion wires well due to the soft tissue envelope. Since a minimum of three points of fixation are needed for optimal stability, an attempt is always made by the author to place four points of fixation (wires alone, half pins alone, or a combination of both) so that if there are problems with one, such as excessive pain or a pin tract infection, it can be removed in the office without compromising the stability of the frame and/or requiring a return to the operating room.

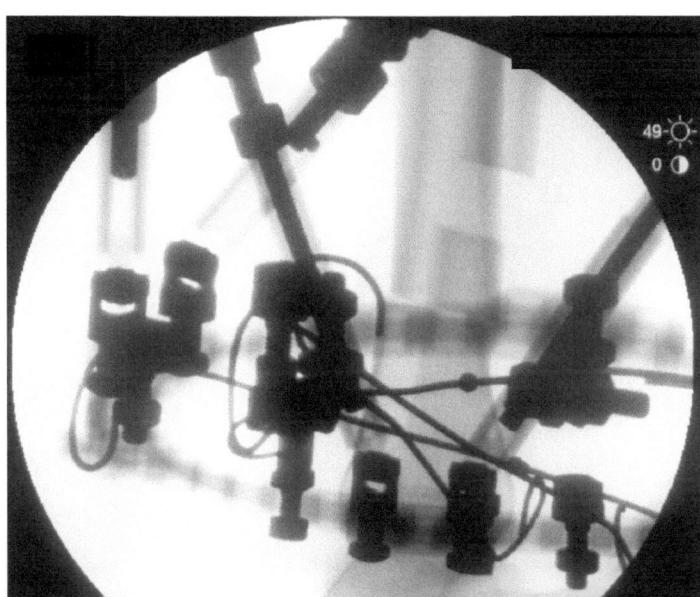

Fig. 23.7 The x-ray beam was positioned for a standard lateral projection of the ankle and not aligned along the axis of the joint, so the ring does not appear appropriately positioned (an oblique projection of the ring is apparent) nor can the tibiotalar joint be seen. The correct orientation of the image intensifier *was* utilized during the case

At this point, the struts connecting the rings were placed and the frame mounting parameters were measured to be later entered into the software program. The corticotomy was then performed using the previously placed Gigli saw (Fig. 23.8). It is important that the frame be absolutely stable prior to performing the corticotomy, especially if a prebuilt frame is used, as the instability created may change the deformity parameters. An additional important point intraoperatively is to be hypervigilant about releasing any tension at all pin sites in whichever direction the skin is noted to be tenting (Fig. 23.9). This helps prevent

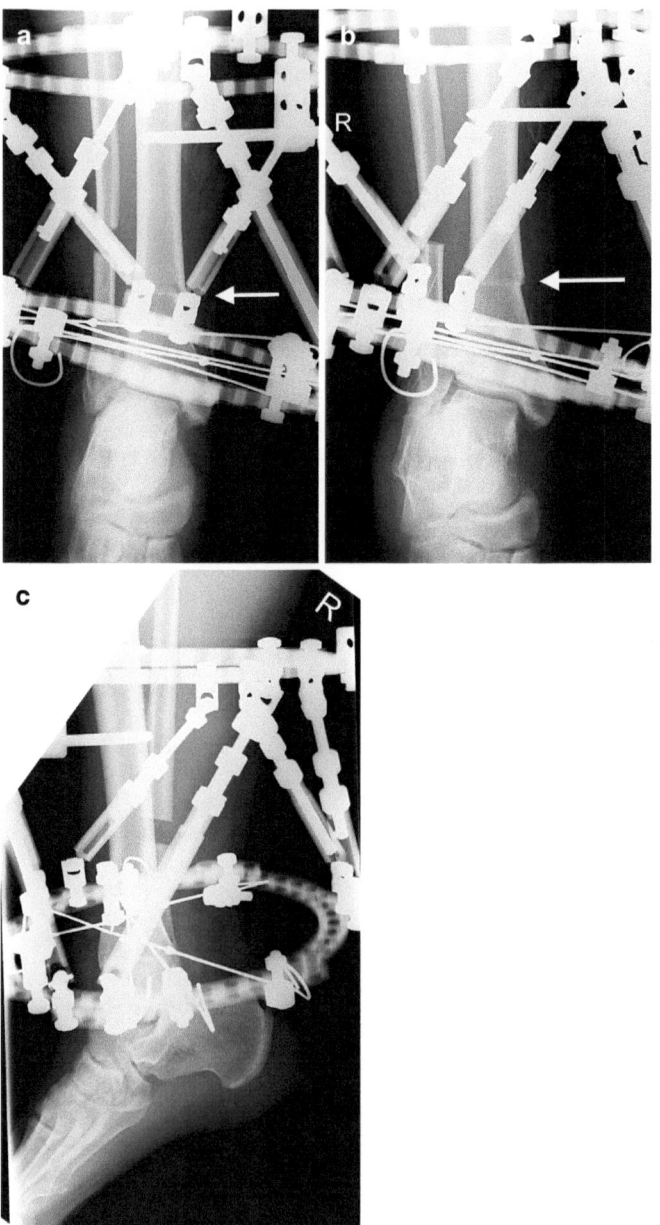

Fig. 23.8 The supramalleolar osteotomy can be seen in the postoperative AP (**a**), oblique (**b**) and lateral (**c**) radiographs

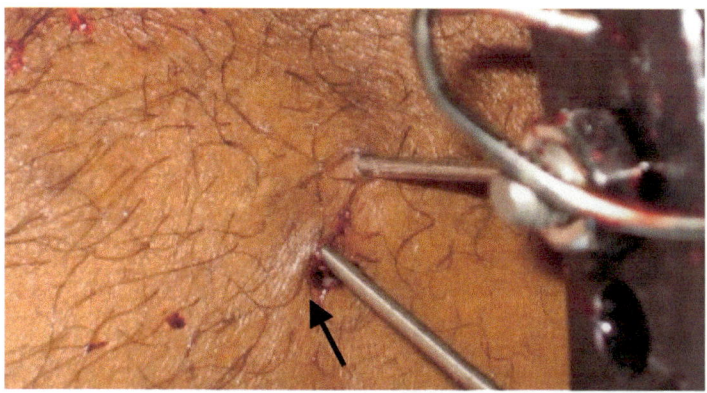

Fig. 23.9 Clinical photograph of a transfixion wire causing tenting of the skin. The skin should be released in the direction of pressure

pressure at the pin-skin interface, which can result in pressure necrosis and contribute to pin tract infections. Pin sites are dressed using specialized sponges held in place by clips that help minimize motion of the skin (Fig. 23.10). These sponges may be silver impregnated to further help prevent pin tract infections. Of note, a fibular ostectomy was also performed in this patient (Fig. 23.11), as an intact fibula could prevent adequate correction of the distal tibia in addition to resulting in disruption of the distal tibiofibular joint. At the conclusion of the case, the appropriate mounting parameters of the external fixator are then entered into the computer program, and the correction schedule is determined (Fig. 23.12).

Postoperative Protocols

When using circular frames for deformity correction, patients are almost always made weight bearing as tolerated immediately postoperatively and this patient was able to actually begin bearing weight on his leg by postoperative day 4. He was ambulating longer distances with a single crutch and around his apartment with no assistive devices after just 2 weeks. By 1 month postoperatively, he was not using any assistive devices.

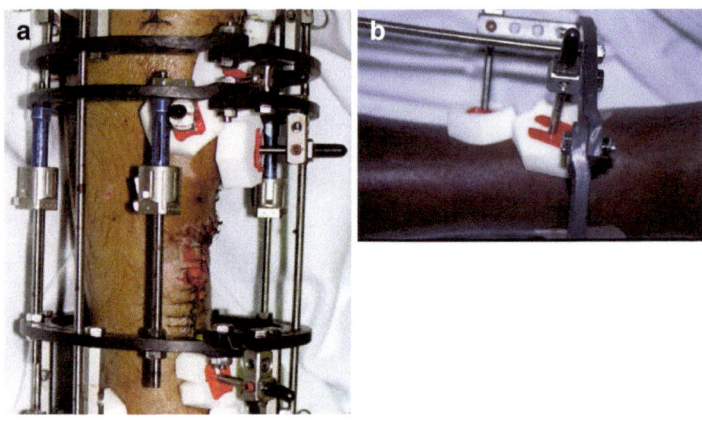

Fig. 23.10 Specialized sponges and clips used to minimize motion at the pin-skin interface (**a, b**)

After a latency period of 7 days to allow completion of the inflammatory process initiated by the corticotomy (typically 7–10 days in adults [3, 4]), the patient began his gradual correction as calculated by the software. He was followed weekly for the first month to ensure patient compliance, appropriate progression of the correction, and to monitor the appearance of the regenerate bone, then biweekly once it was apparent that all was well (Fig. 23.13). Close radiographic follow-up is necessary to make sure there are no problems with the correction, such as the moving segment impinging on the static segment or the creation or a new deformity. This patient did require a revision of his turning schedule at 1 month due to medial translation of the distal tibial segment and procurvatum at the corticotomy site (Figs. 23.14 and 23.15). The remainder of his correction was completed uneventfully with correction of his deformity over the course of 2 months (Fig. 23.16).

Pin care is always an issue with external fixation, as the most common soft tissue complication is pin tract inflammation and/or infection with inflammation rates of up to 100 % reported [5]. There are many recommendations for pin site care with some authors advocating routine low-dose antibiotic therapy throughout the course of treatment in the frame. This author prefers to initially instruct the patient to shower daily with an antibacterial soap,

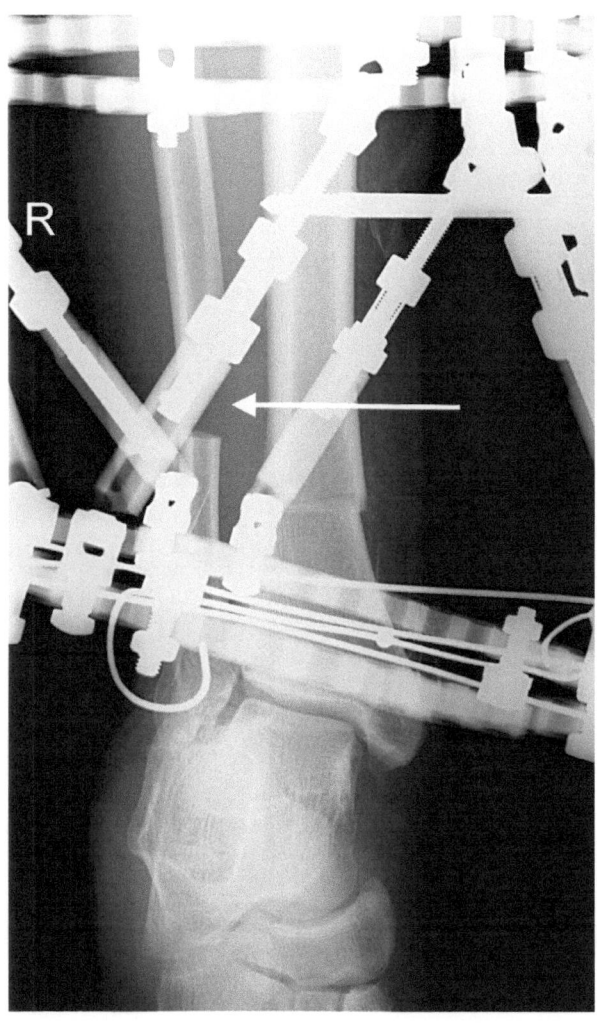

Fig. 23.11 A portion of the fibula was excised (fibular ostectomy) to allow correction of the distal tibia and prevent disruption of the distal tibiofibular joint

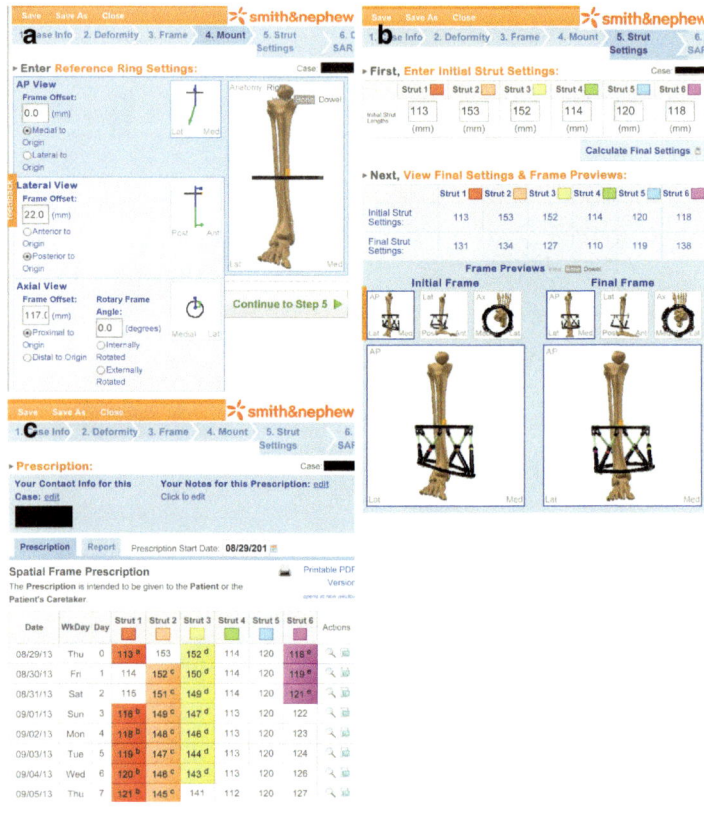

Fig. 23.12 The mounting parameters of the frame are entered into the computer program (**a**) and the program produces a preview of the correction (**b**) as well as a schedule for the patient and surgeon to follow (**c**) (Reproduced with permission: Smith & Nephew, Memphis, TN)

allowing the frame and the leg to get wet. No additional mechanical pin care, such as dilute hydrogen peroxide cleansing of each pin, is initially recommended. The previously illustrated pin sponges and clips can be used on any pin sites with persistent drainage or skin irritation. If the patient continues to have pin site problems, then more aggressive local pin site care will be instituted, reserving the use of antibiotics for failure of local methods.

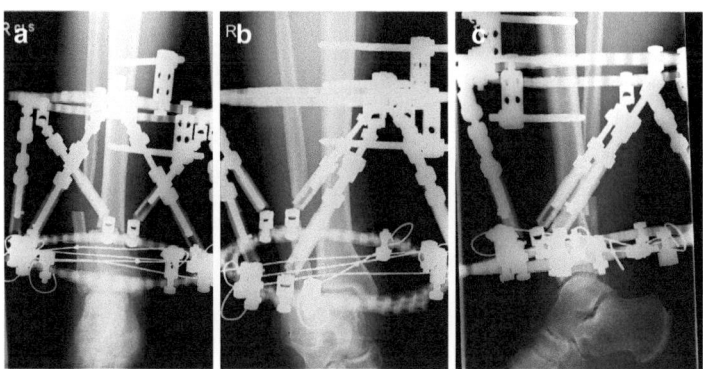

Fig. 23.13 Radiographs obtained after 2 weeks of correction. Movement of the distal tibia can be seen along the medial cortex on the AP (**a**) and oblique (**b**) views. Any changes in the sagittal plane are obscured by the frame (**c**)

If oral antibiotics do not adequately treat the infection, it may be necessary to remove a wire or half pin. Although this patient did require more aggressive local pin care, he did not ever need oral antibiotics. He did develop some nerve irritation from a transfixion wire that coursed near his superficial peroneal nerve over the anterolateral distal tibia after tripping and banging the distal ring of his frame against a solid object; however, his symptoms completely resolved with removal of this wire. Since excess fixation had been placed, it was possible to remove the wire in the office without affecting the stability of the frame.

Follow-Up with Union/Complications

Typically, the consolidation phase for healing of the regenerate bone is at least twice the length of time required for correction of the deformity. For this patient, it took him 2 months to complete his correction, and he wore the frame a total of 6 and a half months until it was felt that adequate consolidation had been achieved (Fig. 23.17). Before considering frame removal, the patient should be ambulating full weight bearing without pain and with limited or no use of assistive devices. Prior to frame removal, it is important

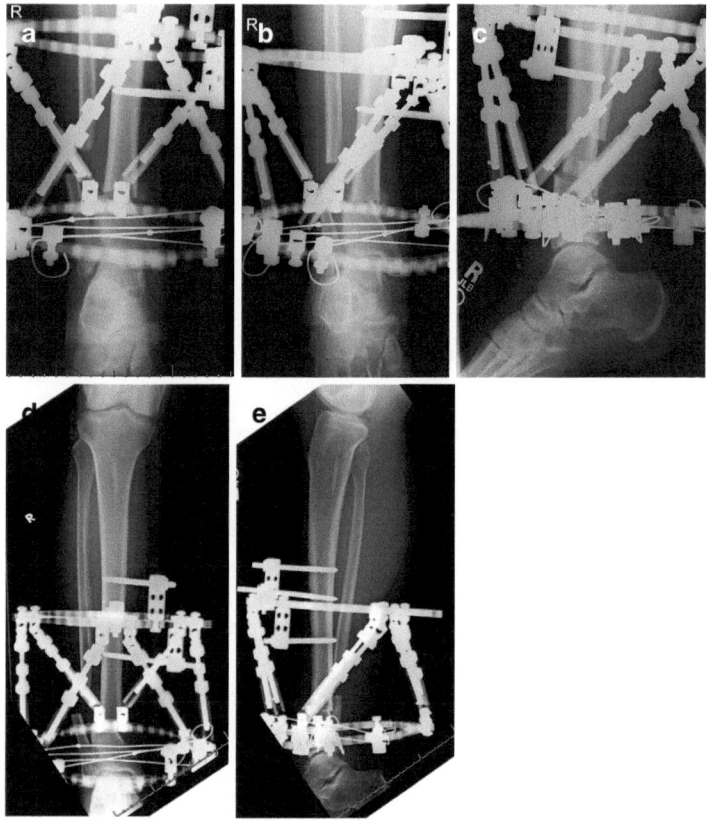

Fig. 23.14 Radiographs obtained after 4 weeks of correction show the creation of medial translation of the distal fragment as seen on the AP (**a**) and oblique (**b**) ankle views as well as on the AP view of the tibia (**d**). A procurvatum deformity is noted on the lateral (**c**) ankle view. This is not seen on the lateral tibia radiograph (**e**) and illustrates the importance of obtaining both ankle radiographs centered over the juxta-articular deformity to identify more subtle deformities as well as full-length tibia radiographs to follow overall alignment

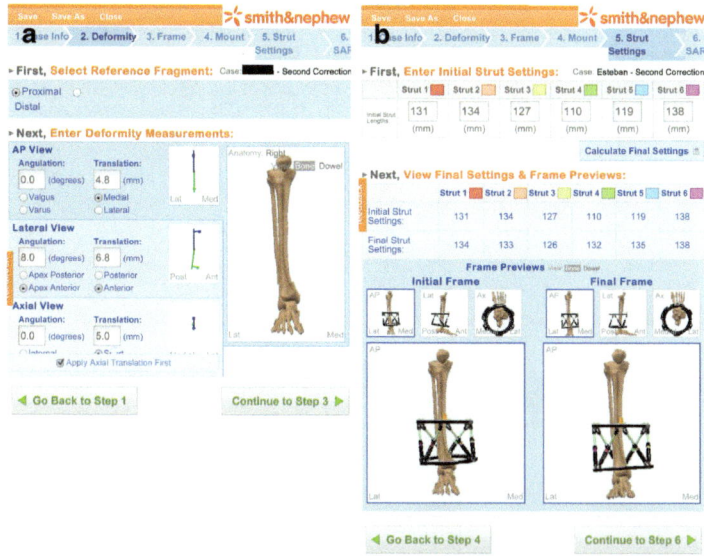

Fig. 23.15 New deformity parameters were entered for a residual correction (**a**) and a new preview of the correction was generated (**b**) along with a new schedule (not shown) (Reproduced with permission: Smith & Nephew, Memphis, TN)

to dynamize or destabilize the frame to ensure that the healed bone is supporting the patient's weight, and not the frame. Multiple oblique radiographs or even a CT scan may be required to assess healing due to the frame frequently obscuring the bone on standard radiographs, although this was not necessary in this patient. Once the patient tolerates dynamization, the frame is then removed. Since the author typically uses hydroxyapatite coated half pins due to the anticipated prolonged wear time of the frame, removal of the external fixator is performed in the operating room under anesthesia. After frame removal, the patient is usually not placed into any type of immobilization and remains weight bearing as tolerated. Continued remodeling of the regenerate bone can be anticipated even after frame removal (Fig. 23.18). Two weeks postoperatively, this patient was walking many miles a day with no complaints. He ambulated with a near normal gait, and was happy with his result but has since been lost to follow-up.

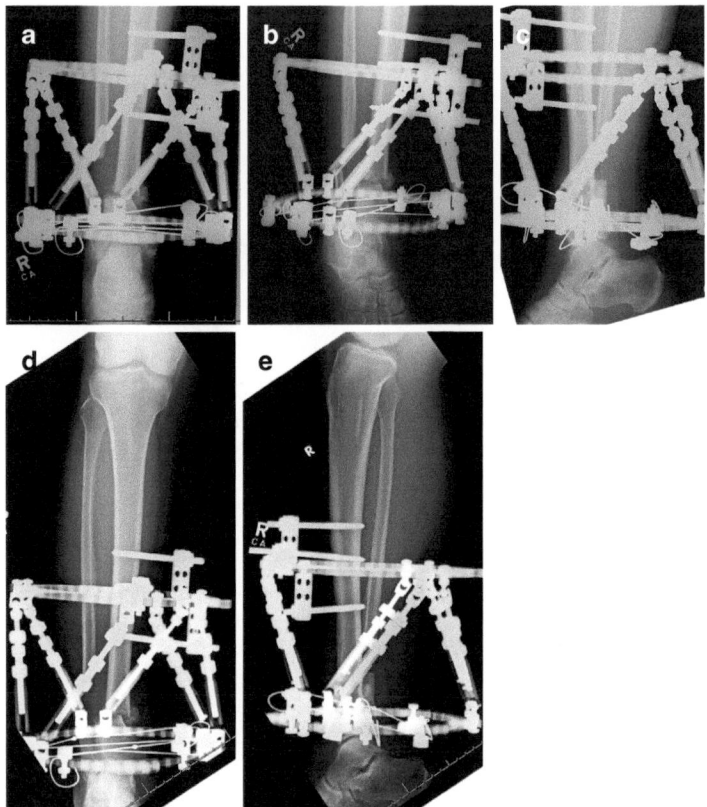

Fig. 23.16 Completion of the correction with early callus formation around the corticotomy site noted (**a**–**e**). Despite the fact that the distal tibia initially appears laterally displaced relative to the shaft (**a**, **b**), the overall alignment shows the talus to be centrally positioned under the plafond in both AP (**a**, **d**) and lateral (**c**, **e**) projections of the ankle and the tibia. Note that both rings now appears nearly as a single line on the AP (**a**) and lateral (**c**) views compared to the oblique appearing position of the distal ring on the lateral view in the initial post-operative radiographs (Fig. 23.8c)

The use of external fixation for treatment of tibial malunions is an excellent option for patients who may have complex multiplanar deformities or juxta-articular deformities that can make uniplanar corrections more difficult. The advent of computer-aided correction has greatly simplified the use of circular ring external fixators for both congenital and

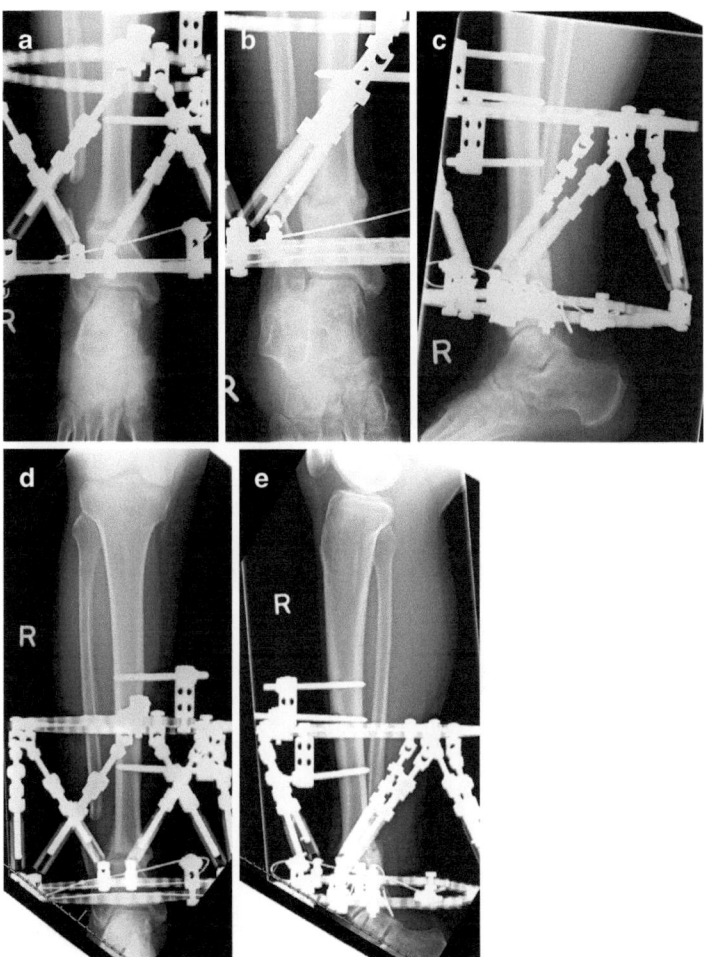

Fig. 23.17 Correction has been maintained and the corticotomy site is fully healed (**a–e**)

post-traumatic deformity correction, but the technique remains technically demanding and is fraught with many potential complications. However, the ability to fine-tune and continuously readjust the correction during the course of treatment makes this a very powerful and predictable technique for treatment of tibial malunions.

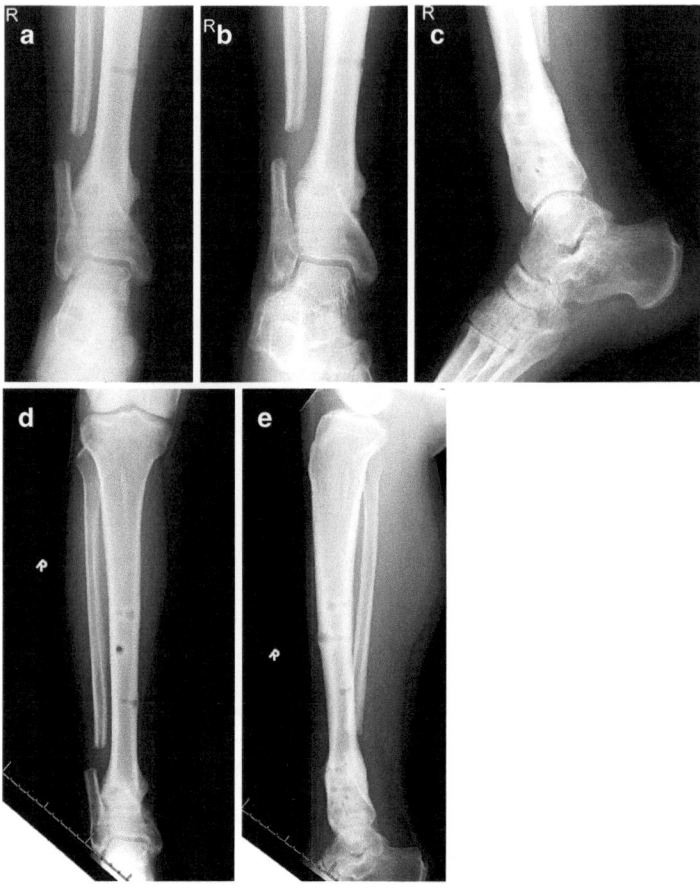

Fig. 23.18 Continued consolidation of the corticotomy site can be seen (**a–e**) after removal of the frame

Pearls/Salient Points

Computer-aided circular ring external fixation is a potent tool for managing complex tibial deformities in carefully selected patients.

- Meticulous preoperative planning, including appropriate imaging *and* management of patient expectations is essential to success.

- Intraoperatively, selection of the appropriate site for the corticotomy and close attention to placement of the rings, transfixion wires, and half pins can help minimize postoperative complications.
- A fibular osteotomy is often required to prevent an intact fibula from blocking correction of the tibia.
- Disadvantages:
  - Technically demanding
  - Requires close patient follow-up to ensure strict compliance to scheduled adjustment of the frame

- Advantages compared to acute correction:

  - Immediate weight bearing
  - Computer-aided ability to continuously adjust and readjust the correction
  - Predictable and reproducible technique in properly selected patients

References

1. Paley D, Tetsworth K. Percutaneous osteotomies. Osteotome and Gigli saw techniques. Orthop Clin North Am. 1991;22(4):613–24.
2. Eralp L, Kocaoglu M, Ozkan K, Turker M. A comparison of two osteotomy techniques for tibial lengthening. Arch Orthop Trauma Surg. 2004;124(5):298–300.
3. Ilizarov GA. The tension-stress effect on the genesis and growth of tissues. Part I. The influence of stability of fixation and soft-tissue preservation. Clin Orthop Relat Res. 1989;238(238):249–81.
4. Ilizarov G. The tension-stress effect on the genesis and growth of tissues: Part II. The influence of the rate and frequency of distraction. Clin Orthop Relat Res. 1989;239:263.
5. Watson J, Anders M, Moed B. Management strategies for bone loss in tibial shaft fractures. Clin Orthop Relat Res. 1995;315:138–52.

Index

© Springer International Publishing Switzerland 2016
N.C. Tejwani (ed.), *Fractures of the Tibia: A Clinical Casebook*,
DOI 10.1007/978-3-319-21774-1